APHASIA

APHASIA

by Arnold Pick

Translated and Edited by

JASON W. BROWN, M.D.
*Assistant Clinical Professor of Neurology
Columbia University
New York, New York*

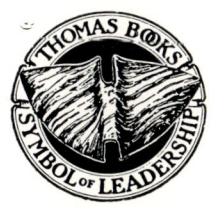

CHARLES C THOMAS · PUBLISHER
Springfield · Illinois · U.S.A.

Published and Distributed Throughout the World by
CHARLES C THOMAS · PUBLISHER
BANNERSTONE HOUSE
301-327 East Lawrence Avenue, Springfield, Illinois, U.S.A.

This book is protected by copyright. No part of it may be reproduced in any manner without written permission from the publisher.

© *1973*, by CHARLES C THOMAS · PUBLISHER
ISBN 0-398-02658-0
Library of Congress Catalog Card Number: 70-169873

With THOMAS BOOKS *careful attention is given to all details of manufacturing and design. It is the Publisher's desire to present books that are satisfactory as to their physical qualities and artistic possibilities and appropriate for their particular use.* THOMAS BOOKS *will be true to those laws of quality that assure a good name and good will.*

This book was originally published as an article by Arnold Pick in the *Handbuch der normalen und pathologischen Physiologie,* Volume 15, published in 1931 by Springer-Verlag, Heidelberg, Germany.

Printed in the United States of America
H-2

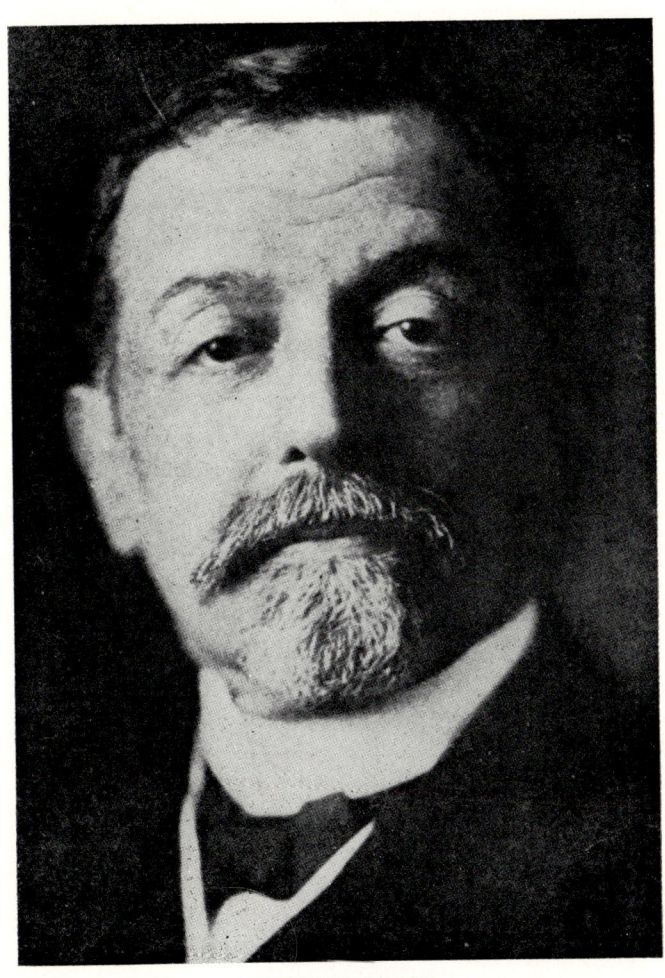

ARNOLD PICK
July 20, 1851 -- April 4, 1924

ARNOLD PICK

ARNOLD PICK was born into a time of awakening Czech nationalism in the aftermath of the 1848 revolution in a small town, Gross Meseritsch (Velké Meziriči), in Moravia. Here and in Iglau (Jihlava) where he went to elementary school and gymnasium, he grew up in a tense bilingual environment. His parents identified with the German enclave and it was only natural that Pick went to the University of Vienna (1869). He came to the capital city of a great empire. The people enjoyed a cosmopolitan culture and passionately indulged with deep devotion in the fine arts, and the medical faculty had a world wide reputation of excellence. Vienna's inspirations and influences left indelible impressions in Pick's personality. He was not a glamour student, yet under the aegis of Hyrtl, Rokitansky and Meynert, adopted a keen view for fine details and a methodical approach to scientific problems. While still a medical student and assistant at Meynert's clinic (1872), he published a scientific essay foreshadowing a promising lifework.

After his graduation (Feb. 12, 1875) he went to Berlin to work in the well-known Charité Hospital under Westphal, who undoubtedly inspired his early interest in spinal cord pathology. At the Charité, he met his contemporary Wernicke, already well known for his work on aphasia. After a brief intermezzo (Dec. 1875 to May 1877) as staff physician at the hospital for mental diseases in Wehnen, Pick accepted a similar position in Prague. Here he received an academic title and a faculty membership as Dozent in Psychiatry and Neurology (June 24, 1878). His clinical work and scientific publications brought him early recognition, and in 1880 he was made director of the Bohemian Irrenanstalt (Hospital for Mental Diseases) Dobran. At the age of 35, he was appointed Professor and Chairman of Psychiatry and Neurology at the German (Ferdinand) University of Prague (July 18, 1886).

He held this position for 35 years, which were by no means always easy. In his own words, Pick recalled that he was "not at all satisfied with numerous unfavorable circumstances" of the psychiatric clinic. An old baroque convent (St. Catherine's) housed the German psychiatric clinic and hospital, of which he was chairman. It was ill-equipped to serve as a hospital, and was deemed only a temporary solution, but the promised new building never materialized. Permanent overcrowding, poor hygienic facilities, lack of equipment and laboratory space, and unending difficulties in hiring sufficient bilingual medical and paramedical personnel, partly stifled his initial enthusiasm. Poor funding cut down many of his research projects. He had to fight constantly against administrative hurdles and bureaucratic chicanery by the provincial (Bohemian) as well as by the central (Austro-Hungarian) government. The simmering political animosity between the German and Czech populace could be felt everywhere. Petty envy and a hostile rivalry between the German (Ferdinand) and the Czech (Charles) Universities were not kept just within academic boundaries all the time. A man with less discipline would have given up soon. Not so Pick, particularly since he found in Otto Kahler a congenial associate in neuropathological research at the German University. Pick's fame as a scientist, his calm personality and political impartiality were of unquestionable importance in preventing his ouster by the postwar independent Czech Government. Although in retirement (Dec. 31, 1921) because of his age and poor health, having lost one eye in 1915 due to complications after retinal detachment, Pick continued an active scientific life and published several of his most important papers on aphasia. Death came suddenly due to postoperative sepsis and cardiac failure.

Pick was always the great universalist, and combined the devotion of the old-line clinician with the compulsive thoroughness and criticism of the researcher and theorist. He was a very demanding chief, requesting his assistants to stay with him long after regular hours or to listen to his seemingly unending interviews of psychiatric patients. Painstaking records, consideration of every detail, and cautious use of data were the most significant criteria of his work as a physician and scientist. Moreover, he was primarily responsible for acquainting German neurology with the teachings of Head, Sherrington, Jackson and Charcot, to name only the most prominent figures. In addition to his well-known work on spinal cord diseases, psychiatric and aphasic disorders, he was also a strong advocate of reforms of the desolate psychiatric systems and institutions of his time. A number of publications in professional journals and the lay press deal with the fundamental humanitarian, social and legal aspects of the mentally sick.

Pick's private life always remained overshadowed by his consuming professional activities as researcher, teacher and physician. He was a great lover of classical music, fine books and cultivated discussions. In his home he preferred a quiet and modest style of life devoted to his family. He attracted many friends among his colleagues, the closest being Otto Kahler, but he maintained contact with many others outside the medical field, mostly well-known personalities in the natural and philosophical sciences. With almost all contemporary European neurologists of note, Pick maintained a lively and mutually rewarding correspondence. His death was mourned well beyond his native country. Though his loss was felt for a long time, he has left behind a rich legacy: a great number of well-trained pupils and associates, and a great body of important and still-relevant writings.

DR. F. STIEGLMAYR

References

1. Sittig, O.: Professor Arnold Pick. *Arch. Psychiatr., 72*:1-20, 1925.
2. Sittig, O.: Professor MUDr. Arnold Pick, *Jahrb. Psychiatr. u. Neurol., 44*:I-X, 1925.
3. Brown, M.R.: Arnold Pick (1851-1924). In Haymaker, W. and Schiller, F.: *The Founders of Neurology.* Springfield, Thomas, 1970.

EDITOR'S INTRODUCTION

I

WITH THE CURRENT resurgence of interest in aphasia and psycholinguistics it is appropriate at this time to make available to an English speaking audience this classical work by Arnold Pick, first published as a chapter in the *Handbuch d. norm. u. path. Physiol.* (vol. 15, pp 1416-1524, 1931). In the prefatory note to the original edition, Rudolf Thiele noted that the original manuscript was completed shortly before Pick's death in 1924, and then prepared for publication by Otto Sittig. Subsequently, Thiele subjected it to close examination and attempted, so far as possible, to smooth out any roughness of form, without disturbing the "unique character of Pick's expository style." Thiele also appended notes to the text, which have been deleted in this edition as they do not contribute greatly to the original discussion.

Although Pick's contributions to neurology were far-ranging, his most brilliant work was unquestionably in the field of aphasia. Here he played a major role in diverting attention away from the simplistic and diagrammatic accounts which proliferated at the time, and redirecting interest in the deeper and more serious problems of language study and brain action. Among these, none was so difficult as the character of linguistic change, its relation to pathological language, and the nature of their correlation to specific brain areas. Pick attacked this problem head-on and his solution is the high-water point of historical research in aphasia. Central to his approach was the attempt to go beyond limited "horizontalist" or mechanistic concepts of language pathology. There was a recognition of the fact that language has a developmental or productive nature, that it passes through a formative, constructive process leading from cognition to articulate speech, and that disorders of language correspond to damage of this process at various stages in its progression. For neurologists, this approach has a special importance. Pick was familiar with work in psycholinguistics and language learning and tried to apply these to the problems of aphasia. Moreover, he was aware of the need for accurate pathological correlation, and hoped to develop an aphasia theory grounded in both pathological and psychological data. This goal was not fully achieved, though he did provide the groundwork for all later attempts in this direction.

Pick conceived the aphasias as manifestations, in the breakdown of language, of otherwise normal stages in its production. The language mechanism was a dynamic, emergent system, anatomically distributed over the "speech axis" of the brain. Processes underlying this mechanism were damaged in aphasia. The anatomical loci to which these processes related, therefore, referred to sequential stages in language production. Accordingly, in the process of language production, the mental content passed from an early stage coextensive with cognition and memory through levels of progressive differentiation on the way toward articulate speech. In this progression the language form developed, by a kind of serial transformation, out of a diffuse spatial core. This led to the formation of a sentence pattern and then to the stages of word choice and phonemic selection. This account of a transition from a spatial or structural phase to a temporal or serial phase gave rise to subsequent attempts to define a spatial deficit in deep level or "thought-close" aphasias, and a temporal deficit in the surface or "word-close" forms. Examples of this are Head's semantic aphasia and Luria's kinetic motor aphasia respectively.

More specifically, Pick noted that the processes of language "do not consist of an assumed collection of 'elements'," but rather, "are from their very beginning patterned structures (Gestalten)." The early phase of language production is embedded in a cognitive matrix out of which the sentence pattern will emerge; the *proposition*, as the unit of speech, will underlie all subsequent forms. Pick described four phases in this transitional process: an early stage (1) in which thought is formulated with increasing clarity out of memory in such a way that its partial contents are combined to a type of schematic or structural whole; this stage (2), that of structural thought, is prior to linguistic formulation; there is a preparation toward a predicative arrangement, and elements of tone, tempo and grammar come in play; the next stage (3), that of a sentence pattern, develops under the influence of an (imprecisely defined) emotional factor, and leads to (4) the automatic choice of words. The intuitive and structural stages of thought development of Pick and later workers, such as Bouman and Grunbaum, are comparable to the Bewusstseinlagen and Bewusstheit of the Würzburg school, and the levels of the sphere and the concept of Paul Schilder.

With regard to "receptive" disturbances, Pick assumed a complementary mental structure underlying the transition of heard sound to thought, and aligned the various pathological categories along this hypothetical frame. Although he did not give to speech comprehension the same constructive activity assumed for expression, his discussion of disorders of auditory attunement or attention acknowledges an awareness of the active nature of perception. By this he seems to have meant a motor focusing on perception, a kind of exploration of the acoustic environment and a fixation upon speech sounds. When this mechanism was damaged, a severe disturbance in language comprehension followed. The mechanism is also discussed in relation to the expressive forms.

Other aspects of Pick's contribution that should be mentioned include his treatment of the "center," and his concept of localization. A "center" corresponds to that anatomical locale which has to do with a particular segment of the emerging linguistic pattern. Localization, therefore, concerns both the identification of "centers" in this sense, and their correlation with stages in the language process. Pick also spoke of a variety of mechanisms, some of which were so correlated, and others not. These include the mechanism of phonemic serialization attributed to the "executive speech organ"; the process of motor focussing, which is comparable to the modern notion of attention and set; and, especially, the role of the feeling for the language, Sprachgefühl, in guiding and organizing the language resources. This latter capacity, unconsciously acquired and specific to the individual language, helps in the ordering of speech, its automatization, naturalness and rhythmicity. Many diverse conditions are referred by Pick to a disturbance of Sprachgefühl, and one cannot help but wish that a more precise characterization were available.

A similar reaction may occur to his discussion of the distinction between consciousness of content and consciousness of action, the reduction of awareness or its uneven distribution over different facets of the speech act, the nature and degree of alignment between certain speech contents and the "transmission apparatus," and so on. Yet, though the treatment is somewhat vague, and employs a mentalistic formulation that is rarely in concert with contemporary attitudes, the very attempt, at times moderately successful, to account for some of these important aspects of our subjective experience will not, it is hoped, fail to impress the reader.

In contrast to this, Pick also tried to specify certain of these phenomena in more physiological terms. One example is his definition of inner speech as "the form of excitation of the motor-speech apparatus that has become habitual for that individual." Another example is the schema of disinhibitory syndromes, in which such diverse conditions as logorrhea and paraphasia were subsumed under a common physiological mechanism. With regard to aphasic symptoms and the various categories of aphasia, the reader is directed especially to Pick's masterly discussion of repetition disorders, of paraphasia and echo-syndromes, and the classical account of agrammatism and the varieties of grammatical disturbance. Finally, the reader's attention is called to the authoritative discussion of the importance of certain "general factors" in aphasia, such as individual differences, education and practise, the variable participation of the minor hemisphere in the symptomatology, compensatory adaptations and fatigue, the action of the "whole" brain in comparison with focal lesions, and the effect of psychic or personality factors on the aphasia type.

II

This translation had its start when, several years ago, I first became aware of this concise summary of Pick's work in aphasia, and recognized the close relationship to avenues of my own thinking. I soon realized also its great value to contemporary neurological thought, not only for the brilliant description of aphasic symptomatology but also for the original and penetrating theoretical point of view. Thus, it seemed important to provide both an accurate translation of the content, as well as, so far as possible, a conveyance of the larger shaping attitudes which figure so strongly in this work. At the present time there is an emphasis, particularly in this country, on theories which are the outgrowth of old "associationist" doctrine. While this translation makes no pretense to be the antidote to this trend, it is hoped, perhaps through reopening the historical debate on these central issues, to at least present its audience with a compelling alternative.

It is a pleasure to acknowledge the cooperation of Dr. James Henry of the Armed Forces Institute of Pathology. His assistance in the preparation of this monograph was no less than providential for the interpretation of the many complex tangles in Pick's thought and style. The manuscript was also reviewed for accuracy of translation by Dr. F. Stieglmayr, who has been kind enough to contribute, from the vantage point of his own background, a biographical sketch of Pick's life and career. The photograph of Arnold Pick is reprinted from *Founders of Neurology* through the kind permission of Dr. Webb Haymaker and Charles C Thomas, Publisher. We are also grateful to J. Springer, Publishers, for permission to publish this work in translation. Finally, I would like to particularly acknowledge the warm assistance and thoughtfulness of Mr. Payne Thomas, who has encouraged us from the start in this undertaking.

Lastly, if I may take the immodest opportunity to provide a dedication to another author's work, I would like this little book to recall to the reader the memory of two great pioneers in aphasia theory, Johannes Nielsen, an extraordinary man and my first teacher of aphasia, and Paul Schilder, whose writings have been of great personal value and whose genius has enriched this field forever.

JASON W. BROWN

CONTENTS

	Page
Editor's Introduction	ix

Chapter

1. INTRODUCTION ... 3
2. DIFFERENTIATION OF TERMS ... 6
3. DEVELOPMENT OF SPEECH IN THE CHILD ... 9
4. FRONTAL APHASIC DISTURBANCES OF SPONTANEOUS SPEECH: SO-CALLED MOTOR APHASIA ... 14
5. UNDERSTANDING OF SPEECH: THE PATH FROM SPEECH TO THOUGHT ... 27
6. THE PATH FROM THOUGHT TO SPEECH ... 31
7. INNER SPEECH, THE TRANSMISSION MECHANISM AND THEIR ANATOMICAL LOCALIZATION ... 35
8. DOMINANCE OF THE LEFT HEMISPHERE, SIGNIFICANCE OF THE RIGHT ... 38
9. GENERAL POINTS OF VIEW TO BE TAKEN INTO CONSIDERATION IN THE INTERPRETATION OF PATHOLOGICAL PHENOMENA ... 41
10. PARAPHASIA ... 53
11. PERSEVERATION ... 63
12. REPETITION AND ROTE SPEECH ... 66
13. WORD AMNESIA (AMNESTIC APHASIA) AND OPTIC APHASIA ... 70
14. AGRAMMATISM ... 76
15. WORD DEAFNESS AND SPEECH DEAFNESS ... 87
16. ALEXIA ... 101
17. AGRAPHIA ... 111
18. ARITHMETICAL AND NUMERICAL DISORDERS ... 122
19. CLINICAL FORMS ... 126
20. GESTURE LANGUAGE ... 129

Chapter	Page
21. Amusia	132
22. Aphasia and Intelligence	135
23. Concluding Remarks	138
Biblography	139

APHASIA

Chapter 1

INTRODUCTION

An account of aphasia within the framework of a manual of normal and pathological physiology must go beyond the description of pathological phenomena and their grouping into clinical types in an attempt to embrace, more fully than before, the *processes,* in order to distinguish pathological and normal happenings from each other or at least to define more clearly the considerations that are necessary for such a dynamic interpretation. It must be an attempt, through an increasingly deeper-penetrating description of phenomenology, to achieve an understanding of the pathological processes and their relationships. It is not possible at the present time to base such an understanding on knowledge of the anatomical, histological, or physiological facts; instead it is our task, based upon a consideration of the phenomena themselves, as derived from clinical psychological observations, and thus through an optimal refinement of symptomatology in so far as this is possible, to facilitate the development of a functional theory in this area. Inasmuch as a large part of the subject is deeply rooted in psychodynamics, while other parts have also a psychic aspect, it is impossible to avoid taking a theoretical stand regarding the body-soul problem. Parallelism comes to be applied here as a useful hypothesis, not only because it enables us to better maintain the necessary separation and delineation of somatic and psychic, but because an advanced clarification of one component, in this case the psychic, must simultaneously benefit the other.

One difficulty lies in the status of the problem itself. It is only recently that seemingly adequate clinical inquiry into the residual capabilities of patients with particular lesions has been abandoned; that the character of the disordered *functions* are being investigated in comparison to the normal. Another difficulty lies in the inadequacy of specialized physiology, which in the matters to be considered here is only concerned with and determined by human pathology. Therefore, if detailed clarification of pathologically altered mechanisms seems out of the question, and if for the time being we find ourselves still in the stage of hypotheses based upon description, a thorough account of individual phenomena seems all the more justified in that every peculiarity of these phenomena opens up new points of view. Then, too, there is a transformation of psychological research which influences a consideration of the problem to be discussed here, especially through the recognition of a nondirected (anschauungslosen) thought and of *gestalt* problems. But the psychological material cannot be completely exploited, since at present the clinical parallels are often either lacking or not yet discovered. We must also take into account the current concept which suggests that from sensory experiences to the highest psychic processes, including speech, we are confronted with an ascending series of functions upon which are superimposed mechanisms of increasing unification (coordination, integration) resulting in sequences ordered in space and time. Furthermore, these processes do not consist of an assumed collection of "elements"; rather they are from their very beginning "patterned structures" (gestaltete Strukturen) which form the basis for those groupings that take place later. It is only through subsequent artificial analysis, occasioned at times by pathological processes, that the assumed "elements" come to be perceived.

This reorientation is in contrast to the old theory of aphasia which dealt primarily with "memory images contained in the respective centers." Yet it also appears to be justified by similar views which are becoming established in speech psychology and linguistics. Because biology and the general physiology of the brain are also affected by the same new orientation, they match the "structures" and *"gestalten"* of the psychologists with their own "schemata," "patterns," and the like.

Such a functionally based dynamic conception, holding aloof from any attempt to go beyond the empirical and set up those formulations derived as correct, is the starting point for an attempt at a theory of aphasia more far reaching than earlier ones. On the other hand, we cannot conceal the fact that such an attempt can find only limited support from anatomical and physiological correlates, the knowledge of which has not yet advanced so far. Despite the unfinished state of the material, and despite the brevity of the presentation and the impossibility of critical comparison with conflicting views, the attempt to develop such a theory appears justified by the clear evidence of the gaps in our knowledge and the necessity of deriving an understanding of insights already attained. Various special aspects that modify the conception of aphasia will be presented in the general discussion below. At this point, let us merely add a note on the nomenclature. When "centers" are spoken of, the word is intended to denote only the functionally most prominent and consequently not sharply delimitable part of a system of structural relationships which corresponds to an increasingly refined degree to developing functional systems (not the seat of a particular faculty, not even in the physiological sense of a preformed apparatus associated with sharply circumscribed functions). A lesion of such a "center" (including functional lesions) disturbs most easily the more prominent capacities while related functional groups may also be disturbed in varying degree. This means that collections of neurons united in such a center, and functions associated with them, can also be selectively impaired. While we thus seem on the way to a *localization of function,* such a conception as this does away with the necessity of creating a specific center for every disorder, a need for which the older theory has been criticized. For this reason, we avoid setting up a diagram to clarify the various aphasic disorders, as it would go beyond the thesis presented here and fix the imprecisely known localizations, as well as the unknown but postulated connecting paths between the various centers. All such attempts at systematic explanation disguise the complexity of the reality, to which no comprehensible diagram could do justice. In this respect, it is worth noting that in the past it was precisely that which was regarded as established, fixed in the diagram, and apparently best explained which turned out to be most obscure and in need of explanation.

Chapter 2

DIFFERENTIATION OF TERMS

Corresponding to the double nature of speech as a sequence of tones and noises (or the written symbols corresponding to them) culminating in the *patterned* expression of intellectual content, we distinguish the primary motor disturbances (of voice, articulation, [anarthria] and writing) and the corresponding disorders of hearing and sensation from those collectively grouped as aphasic. The latter are disorders which, although not determined by mental disturbances in the narrow sense of the word, effect speech in its capacity as an expression of mental activity. That which is spoken, heard, seen as symbols for what is thought and felt, Kant's *facultas signatrix,* achieve a formulation in speech symbols. To the same field belong the functions of gesture and, to a lesser extent, those of mimic and music—disturbances of which will also be discussed.

The delimitation given here also corresponds to that which has prevailed recently in linguistic science: (1) The science of sounds (phonology), (2) the science of meaning (semiology [Noreen], semasiology or semantics), and (3) morphology. If the latter is the science of the forms in which the phonic material is shaped to the purpose of representing meaning, it is evident that the subject of aphasia embraces the pathology of both semiology and morphology and cannot even entirely dispense with phonology, insofar as it is concerned with the conveyance of meaning. It is understandable that pathological morphology has been relatively best worked out. The gaps in our knowledge are particularly evident in the field of semiology. As a suggestion for further studies, let me point out that this shortcoming is attributable in no small part to the fact that the clinical stage best suited to the study of semantic disorders—namely that of improvement or outward cure of the various aphasias where the disorders of style, no longer obscured by disorders of speech or writing are particularly evident—has as yet been little studied for our purposes, largely because this stage of restitution has been incorrectly regarded as no longer belonging within the framework of the aphasias.

As opposed to this sharp differentiation according to motor, sensory, and psychic aspects, and in view of the close relationships between the functional areas in question, it will not infrequently happen that disorders of these categories are present as a part of one or another form of aphasia. Moreover, because of the inadequacy of our diagnostic tools, there will often be difficulties, partly because disorders of one area may first appear in the dysfunction of another subordinate or related area. On the psychic side, we must consider the fact that in the execution of impressionally excited thought and in thought being prepared for expression, disturbance of the latter may become apparent, while on the other hand a sharp distinction between sensation and perception, and their disorders, is hardly possible. With respect to the demarcation on the psychic side, Head especially has emphasized that certain forms of aphasic disorders are only a partial expression of more extensive mental disorders that extend beyond verbalization. It is also consistent with these observations that pure cases of the "schemas" become progressively more rare. Deeper research discloses finer differences in what appear to be clinically similar modes of behavior, with the result that practical and scientific appraisals often differ in individual cases. It is further in accord with this that the traditional terms—aphemia, agraphia, word-deafness—no longer do justice to the phenomena except in the crudest and clinically barely adequate degree.

The cohesive system of linguistic means available for the expression of the psychic is associated with a multitude of physiological functions, for the execution of which a system of cerebral organs has developed. These stand in an integrative relationship to each other; anatomically, they constitute the speech center, which together with the functionally interrelated field of musical functions embraces the greater part of the area surrounding the fissure of Sylvius, including the greater part of the Insula (Fig. 1); a second region partially surrounding this one and largely including the temporal lobes, with as yet poorly defined borders, may be regarded in relation to those functions which mediate psychic phenomena in the stricter sense. To what extent extrapyramidal and cerebellar functions, as is likely, are also involved in

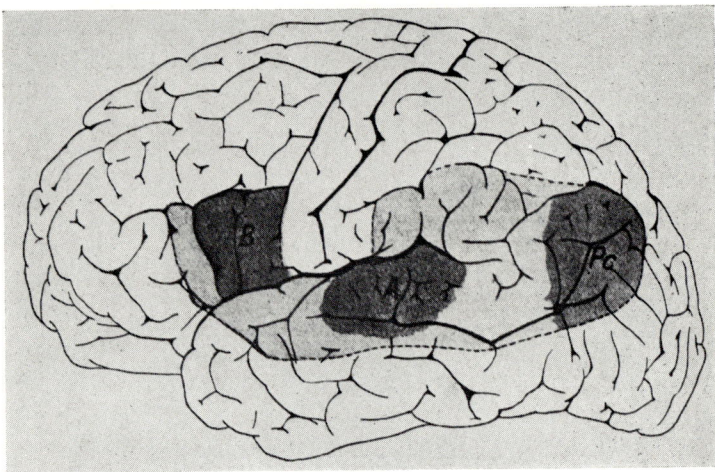

Figure 1. The speech zone: B = Broca's convolution. A = Wernicke's convolution. Pc = Angular gyrus. (from Dejerine, 1914.)

certain motor components of speech (rhythm, accent) analogues with other forms of motion has not yet been fully determined.

The fact that the expressive functions of the speech field are principally in its frontal portion, while the impressive sensory functions are in the temporal part, corresponds to the *classification of aphasias* into *frontal* and *temporal*. The latter designation is preferable to the old one of "sensory aphasias," since sensory disturbances are often lacking (or at any rate, not prominent) while disorders of expression may often have their basis in temporal lesions.

Chapter 3

DEVELOPMENT OF SPEECH IN THE CHILD

A KNOWLEDGE OF the development of speech is indispensable for the understanding of numerous facts of pathology. Speech normally takes its origin, after a certain degree of intellectual development is attained, from the presence of the normal development of the bilateral acoustic centers and of the psychomotor centers of speech; the latter, while perhaps preformed even in the embryonic anlage, certainly continue to develop in the manner of a *conditioned reflex* between the two. The development of speech perception, which precedes the development of active speech by a certain interval, may be characterized as follows: from the diffuse consciousness background of the infant, which arises from the most varied sensory impressions, certain acoustic impressions come to be accentuated because of the feelings that accompany them. Among these acoustic impressions, certain musical elements of speech (speech melody, accent) are in the foreground and can be shown for this reason, as well as for their extraordinary persistence in pathological cases, to be established very early. These are gradually joined by affect-laden sound fragments, reinforced by educational drill, from the wider generalized total acoustic environment of the child. The acoustic impressions (acoustic structures) which correspond to these at first consist of whole speech-groups, sentences, which are followed by words (as one-word sentences), with the phonetically most prominent parts of the sentences being gradually sorted out. It is only much later, sometimes not until school education begins, that the individual phonemes (some sixty in number on the average) that make up the words come to be perceived in isolation. Step-by-step with this development there is gradual differentiation of individual impressions, especially optical, from the diffuse total impressions previously present in the other sensory areas. Through an association of these auditory impressions, regularly reinforced by drill, recognition of auditory impressions and their significance advances.

A feature of this phase that deserves special mention, since it is enlightening for the understanding of certain facts of amnestic aphasia, is that terms designating purpose and object usage frequently precede the actual names of the objects. (This is perhaps related to the better visual perception of motion; cf. also onomatopoeic designations. Many linguists date the development of speech from the seeing and hearing of objects in motion). In the early stage of expressive speech development the instinctive, at first almost entirely undifferentiated, motor effects of the most varied sensations and feeling-impressions, initiate the utterances grouped together in the *crying and babbling period,* which, since their results bring pleasure and so are conducive to repetition, serve simultaneously as trial movements for the exercise and development of the speech organs in the direction of motor structure formations. Their predominantly interjectional form makes the great importance of the musical components of speech understandable, as well as their later resistance to damage. By way of a conditioned reflex developed from the instinctive utterances, certainly beginning during that period but not noticeable until the *ensuing phase of infantile echolalia,* there develops an increasingly refined transfer of the acoustic "structures", developed in the receptive organ, to the speech apparatus. In this way, corresponding motor structures, "movement melodies", come to be formed in the speech apparatus as a basis for reproduction, the musical components being followed by the other phonetic components in order, first in relation to affective utterances still produced by reflex, the single word as an expression of the whole situation. Thus, the *expressive sounds* gradually develop into a *communicative sequence of sounds.* Training of the executive speech apparatus on the basis of this auditory motor transference consists in the progressively improved modification of those motor structures derived from the total acoustic impression for the purpose of converting them into that succession of finely-graded automatic motor impulses used in the highly modified sequences of voluntary speech.

During these phases, the development of a higher, intellectual level of function, with concommitant subordination of the previously dominant reflex arc is completed. It is from these levels that *voluntary* activation of the developed motor speech mechanisms takes place, and it is at this level that the strengthening (Erstarken) and *coherence* of their function occurs. This is responsible for the *inhibition* of the primitive reflex, which, in the normal individual, is only rarely perceived thereafter, when, in certain disorders, it is freed from inhibition and appears in the crudest manner. The feelings of pleasure connected with the target objects, together with the enjoyment attached to the increasing improvement of voluntarily initiated speech movements, leads to a union of the two and to a gradual automatization of the entire process. The development of speech comprehension, which has advanced to an understanding of terms of the sentence, is accompanied by a similar development in the expressive sphere (voluntary use of one or two-word sentences; later, the at first affectively regulated ordering of uninflected words; then, but still without schooling, on the basis of analogy with the feeling for the language [Sprachgefühl], for the customary word order, inflection, and sentence formation, the *grammatization of speech* takes place). Superimposed upon the progressively developed complex and inter-related acoustic and motor aspects of the speech apparatus, are added, in conjunction with training in *reading* and *writing*, the optical and motor structures subserving these purposes. Together these constitute what is termed "inner speech", within which, corresponding to development, the acoustic-motor transmission mechanism continues to play the leading role. The anatomical substrate for the previously described functional structure is assumed to lie in corresponding groupings of finely-regulated neurons. It is easier to understand in this way the variety of isolated elements and combinations of dynamic groups than through the assumption of the transmission of engrams and new formation of centers or pathways. The level of childhood performance, when viewed in this fashion can be understood from the extraordinary plasticity of the child's brain.

Representation of the process of speech development as a superstructure over a primary reflex arc affords an opportunity to extend this concept to Sherrington's "final common pathway" which, though as yet only hinted at, by means of this classification permits a more promising interpretation of the physiological substrate than previous theories. The partially outmoded comparison of the speech apparatus with a piano with its registers and pedals now seems more in harmony with the physiology of the motor centers of the cortex, considered "masters" with afferent functions that play upon the cortex, and for which specific neural arrangements for movements of the speech musculature have been recognized (Graham Brown).

With regard to the problem of *learning to read*, a distinction must be made between reading aloud as such and reading with comprehension. While the former may be done through spelling or, better, phonetically, with little consideration of the context of the words, it has the initial affect of developing a fixation of visual forms in the memory embracing first individual words and later whole groups of words, and associating them with the equally uniform and still developing motor-speech patterns. In this process, the auditory forms which correspond to the hearing of what has been read aloud, in part familiar and in part developed in the process itself, assume their role in the transmission process as described above in the development of speech. This is in harmony with the theoretically important fact that written (printed) speech is "second hand" in nature. This association, however, is retarded by reading through spelling, which is often still practiced, to the extent that words and word groups perceived previously as units and produced the same way in speech are reduced into artificial units (letters and syllables). Thus, it is only through a combining of the phonemes into words that a complete assimiliation of the previously practiced acoustic and motor-speech structures is accomplished. But spelling out has a favorable aspect insofar as isolated phonemes are combined into the automated speech melodies and are thus mobilized for new recombinations. The division of words into syllables, however, is the concern of the school or of research.

The automatization of these relationships then rapidly takes place, and with the progressive development of both optical and motor structures, the assistance provided by the acoustic component moves further into the background. Comprehension of content develops along with reading ability. With regard to known "objects", comprehension is conveyed by the accompanying words. Otherwise, comprehension takes place through optical or other sensory representation. The meaning of the sentence, in its relation to sentence content, is understood on the basis of the familiar in meaningful speech and auditory comprehension.

In accordance with this course of development, by means of which, in the skilled reader, the sequence of sounds is drawn directly from what is visually perceived and understood, ordinarily without the conscious aid of the sound of the words (i.e. spelling-out), it is clear that the less-skillful reader will use audible or inaudible vocalizations to understand what he reads. In this instance, and even more clearly in the aphasic, the word sound of inner speech is an "aid", the loss of which is a serious disturbance.

Along with speech, *learning to write* begins with the imitation of written symbols and ends with the development of the corresponding motor structures. The action of these motor structures is controlled by kinesthetic patterns (schemata, as before), which are formed in the process. Initially, this is accomplished volitionally for each individual motion. Subsequently, there is a rapid development and automatization of increasingly more stable motor structures and a patterned grouping of words and larger groups. In certain occupations, (typing, telegraphy), this goes even beyond the sentence. Orthography comes as a final achievement. In spontaneous writing also, after development is complete, the importance of letters perceived and later visualized recedes entirely into the background. The same is true of the sound component of inner speech, through which conversion of thought into serial writing movements initially took place (also here the fact that writing is "second hand" speech).

The extent to which early reading aids will be abandoned depends on the level of skill attained. The reversion to the childhood stage is often quite obvious in pathological cases. But the methods of learning employed by the patient with his residual functions should not be simply equated with the child(!).

The writing of meaningful sentences develops through expressive speech, which is further advanced with the full cooperation of hearing and reading. The culmination of this development appears with the increasingly automatized association of the writing movements in immediate correspondence with the thought content, and the consequent marked reduction of attention effort devoted to the movements. It should also be mentioned that this last observation, that the major part of the attention is directed toward the sense of the discourse, or to that which is written or read, applies also to other speech functions.

Chapter 4

FRONTAL APHASIC DISTURBANCES OF SPONTANEOUS SPEECH: SO-CALLED MOTOR APHASIA

In accordance with the purpose of the Handbook, the following presentation of aphasic disturbances is not oriented according to clinical syndromes. The separation of symptom groups is noted through the insertion of references where necessary.

The manifestations of disturbed spontaneous speech, in respect of its general nature and its symptomatology, are differentiated into initiative, reactive and imitative forms, differing as to whether the lesion is situated in that part of the speech field embracing the foot of F3 and the anterior part of the Insula, or in the temporal region, including T1, posterior Insula, and most of T2 and T3. Accordingly, we speak of *motor-aphasic, frontal* disorders, in which quantitative defects predominate and *"sensory" aphasic, temporal* disorders which are characterized by qualitative defects.

In the former type spontaneous speech may be so impaired that the patient is totally unable to utter a sound, (aphonia, very rare) or can utter only single speech sounds (i.e. only vowels or single consonants). Much more common are cases in which, after an interval of time, single syllables (si, djon) or senseless sequences of syllables, the patient's own or another name, yes or no, or other fragments constitute all that the patient has at his disposal. However, even these cannot be employed at will or in appropriate context. Later, it may become possible for the patient to use these remnants voluntarily and with correct intonation and rhythm (aphemia). Still later, speech will be slow, hesitant, and with choppy intonation. In the early stage, the effort to speak is accompanied by arbitrary positions of the mouth. The spread of these movements over the speech musculature may distort the articulatory structure of individual words to the point of unintelligibility. At the same time, there are often apraxic phenomena in the corresponding regions with inability to show the tongue or the teeth and so on. (Froeschels, 1918; Pick, 1906, 1918, 1919, 1923; Stauffenberg, 1918).

In the early stage of recovery, there may also be poor articulation of certain sounds, e.g. gutteral sounds, and disorders of phonation and breathing. It is noteworthy that even in later stages those phonemes and fragments which are correctly pronounced cannot be produced separately (e.g. forename and surname as a unit, but not the surname by itself). Occasionally, in the early stage, it is possible to reproduce the whole, or at least a part, of the words of a song correctly by means of a more or less correct melody, rendered spontaneously or through imitation. Similarly, in this early stage, polyglots may be able to speak correctly in one of several previously-known languages (usually the mother tongue). In contrast to these severe and often permanent disorders, there are cases in which the symptoms disappear, occasionally with surprising rapidity, through a stage of early agrammatism, to be described later (in cases caused by trauma or surgical intervention, symptoms may disappear after 8 to 10 days). On the other hand, there are cases in which the whole condition extends over a long period, even years, with slow improvement. Both forms of recovery, but especially the former with rapidly improving pronunciation and expanding vocabulary, go through an early stage of one-word sentences. Following this, the patient can soon produce, in normal syntax, sequences of uninflected nouns and verbs. However, the words of grammatical function are dropped, although sentence intonation is often correct. The genesis of this condition lies in the motor sphere, and it is, therefore, referred to as motor agrammatism (telegraphic style, Negersprache). Sometimes there are also admixtures of defective grammatization, incorrect use of prepositions and the like; wrong syntax (such as placing the verb at the end of the sentence) seems to be quite rare; sometimes the inability to utter the right word compels a change in the ongoing sentence construction. Occasionally, disturbances corresponding to the two forms of expressive agrammatism occur side by side but clearly separated: in spontaneous speech the linguistic poverty of the telegraphic style is evident, while in reading aloud or repetition, an improvement occurs due to the imitative effect, although diverse paragrammatisms occur because of inadequate feeling for the language (Sprachgefühl, see page 79).

Agrammatism also occurs in chronic cases where the picture usually is dominated by the motor disturbances (hesitation, distortion of letters, sometimes resulting in stutter-like forms), with impaired intonation and occasional monotone, in striking contrast to the otherwise undisturbed speech melody. The flow of speech in such patients generally depends on the degree of speech impediment, but even in improved cases it is usually abnormal. In the pauses due to the difficulty there are usually expletives or fragments of expletives. In progressive causes, hesitant speech and a slight stutter may represent the prelude to more serious symptoms. In cases which run a favorable course, the phenomena of defective syntax and grammar gradually recede, with a reduction in the slowness and difficulty of the entire speech process with occasional full recovery. In such cases, slight impediments or stylistic lapses may persist which are noticeable only to the patient or his intimate associates. In rare cases, a permanent stutter is the only remaining symptom. Cases of complete aphonia in which the emotional situation elicits certain oaths or even an entire sentence appropriate to the situation, which could never occur at will, must be regarded as reactive. This class of utterance also includes the phenomenon mentioned above of the ability to complete the lyrics of a song following initiation by the examiner, and this provides a transition to rote speech (see below), which may be intact in patients with severe impairment of voluntary speech.

Parenthetically, we should mention, as a rarer phenomena, the disorder which since Coen has been called *Horstummheit* (audimuditas). It is charatcerized by the presence of normal hearing, an unimpaired speech mechanism and adequate intelligence, with failure of speech development, or rudimentary speech. Another rare phenomenon also observed in connection with non-aphasic disorders is mirror speech (Spiegelsprache), which consists of the patient's spontaneous speaking or reading words backwards, either regularly or intermittently, so that the letters either of whole words or of syllables follow each other in reverse order. These cases probably represent displacements of a motor nature, which may appear in various other forms as well (e.g. reverse writing) and also as a visual defect. A similar phenomena often occurs in typical motor aphasia affecting individual words. Much more uncommon still is the speech disorder called *linguistic puerilism* (perhaps better infantilism), which involves all or parts of speech, and is characterized by the fact that the pronunciation of letters is similar, in severe cases identical, to that of the babbling stage of infancy. Suggestions of this are also found in motor aphasia. This phenomena forms a transition to cases, also very rare, which may be designated as *modification of the character of the language*. In this disorder, e.g. Czech becomes Polonized or French Germanized. Similarly, but relatively more common, are cases in which the speech of the aphasic exhibits a dialectal or other coloring, corresponding more or less to the language spoken by the patient before acquiring a later one (e.g. a German's English, spoken perfectly before his illness, thereafter has a German accent).

The discussion of the disorders considered here will have to be based upon the pure cases without greatly disturbed articulation; the interpretation of their dependence on the causal lesion will be based on a description of the process of speech development and the passage *from thought to speech*.

We have seen how physical processes corresponding to the simultaneous awareness of meaningful thought formulated as inner speech, are converted through Broca's area by means of a gradually developed inner speech transfer apparatus into motor sequences which are modulated in accordance with the intonational pattern.

This is achieved by a successive adaptation of the motor structures developed in the executive organs as unconscious movement habits of means of "inner speech", as a kind of coordination of the motor centers by the controlling motor-speech center, while the regulation of articulatory processes in the motor executive organ itself comes chiefly from kinesthetic patterns. If the motor-speech center must be called upon for the initiation and elaboration of sequences in the motor centers of the lowest part of Ca (precentral gyrus), then a lesion of Broca's area (ordinarily in the left hemisphere) will interrupt or seriously impair this process; the patient has, as we say, motor aphasia.

If we first consider the disorders under consideration quite unprejudiced by any theoretical models, they fall into two groups: those in which spontaneous speech and, in severe cases, automatic speech as well are suppressed entirely or with the exception of a few remnants; and those cases in which speech is more or less impeded (disregarding those cases complicated by anarthria or dysarthria). We may then consider the extent to which these disorders can be explained on the basis of the view of the speech process presented here.

For the first group, we find that the basic disorder affects the initiation and conduction of processes in the executive organ. Since a remnant of automatic initiation is still detectable in the majority of cases, the voluntary act or the disturbance of voluntary initiation and continuance of the act of speaking, may be regarded as the essential element. This is proven by various phenomena seen in such patients. First, there is frequently a contrast between the relative ease of involuntary speech and the difficulty with a volitional speech impulse, noticed by the patients themselves; they complain of an inability to convert known words into sounds. Secondly, there is the observation that the inability to begin a word can be aided through repeating the alphabet, by supplying a simple cue (embolophasia), and especially, by the fact that the entire speech act can often be elicited through singing or repetition.

The same basic situation occurs in those cases where the patient speaks whole words but not certain parts of them, or vice versa; in these cases the patient cannot voluntarily break down the movement patterns corresponding to the words and recombine them, as in the normal case, in order to form similar words and word-combinations. Nor is he able to modify words properly as seen in the phenomenon of rote speech to be discussed later, for in this instance the patient can successfully recite an entire list of words, but if interrupted, cannot resume at the same point without returning again to the beginning.

We see a similar phenomenon in the above-mentioned contrast between correct spontaneous speech and the unsuccessful, letter-by-letter quality of voluntary speech; in the latter, of course, the attention directed toward the act causes it to deteriorate still further.

In cases of polyglottism with e.g. aphemia for a later language and retention of a mother tongue, besides the factor of greater automatization in the use of the mother tongue, the factor of impaired adaptation to the other may also play a role, as manifested by the fact that this impediment can be overcome by one of the above-mentioned mobilization aids.

These and other facts which reflect the contrast between volition and automatization indicate that we are not dealing with a disturbance of a "movement plan" (assumed by Liepmann). Rather, such cases as we have discussed prove that neither the motor structures which develop through speech practice nor their corresponding neuronal connections are disturbed. The occurrence of such undisturbed functions as reading aloud, repetition and writing, in the presence of intact inner speech, shows that the defect concerns only the adjustments associated with these functions on the part of the transmission mechanism and processes corresponding to those adjustments. Since memories cannot be stored in movements, the relevant factor of memory must be interpreted in the sense that reactive structures develop which respond to a succession of stimuli with corresponding reaction patterns, and it is this process that is disordered here.

This account of the major part of these disorders cannot of course eliminate the objection that at the time when those processes figuring in the explanations are demonstrable, the "other" hemisphere has already become involved in the recovery. There are cases where the opposition between volition and automatization is demonstrable from the beginning, so that it seems justified to assume an initial diaschisis in those cases where the opposition appears later. That the argument is also valid for those cases in which the right Broca's center participates in the speech act from the beginning is clear without further comment.

In support of this interpretation, we may also cite the fact that the opposition between volition and automatization is now used to explain certain phenomena of movement in paralyzed extremities.

In order to bring the opposition between volition and automatization into harmony with the anatomical facts, it has been assumed (H. Jackson and recently Henschen) that automatic speech is a function of the right hemisphere (in right-handed persons). But (1) this assumption does not agree with the various chronological modalities of clinical behaviour described here, (2) there is nothing known in the pathology of the right hemisphere to support this theory, and (3) nothing that we know about the general relationship between volition and automatization in respect of the corresponding motor organs indicates such a division.

The second group of disorders, those in which speech is possible but quantitatively and qualitatively impaired, can be explained on the basis of a disorder in the previously discussed transmission mechanism which activates the relationships between sensory and motor systems. Here the production of ordered processes in the continuous serial transmission between these systems is involved. The correct sequence of letters and words depends on the correct sequence of individual processes in the transmitting apparatus. This better explains those disorders described by Bonhoeffer as literal paraphasic than does his assumption of the loss of an image of the microstructure of the word.

We must also bear in mind, as a source of general difficulty, the fact that the previously adequate, although curtailed rudimentary and "stationary" volition used during normal speech, is now compromised due to the increased difficulty of execution and becomes vulnerable to numerous impulses affecting the initiation of the process.

It is hardly possible to say anything more specific concerning the precise localization and nature of these disorders. With reference to the temporally conditioned paraphasic phenomena, it should be noted that apart from the important diagnostic factor of tempo, at times retarded, at other times accelerated, we find similarities in sounds produced which result from pronunciation difficulty.

In an attempt to understand motor aphasic disorders great weight has been placed (especially by Dejerine) on the presence or absence of "inner speech," and an attempt has been made to utilize this feature in differential diagnosis. Apart from the uncertainty of such evidence, it has been shown that in identical cases inner speech either may be present or absent, so that we cannot regard it as a factor common to all cases and of causal significance. Certainly, the loss of inner speech, or change in its structural relationships, or any disturbance of the otherwise finely tuned adjustment between inner speech and the motor executive apparatus will have just as damaging an effect as lack of facilitation of the latter. The fact that polyglots retain the ability to comprehend a language that they cannot speak while correctly speaking another, such that their inner speech component must be maintained by the hearing, indicates that loss of inner speech is not the cause of inability to speak; rather, loss of speech represents failure of activation of the corresponding motor structures, at times only those employed in the corresponding *voluntary* function. The various degrees of involvement of inner speech are demonstrated by disorders of reading and writing which accompany the disorders of speech and which would not be expected to occur with isolated defects of the motor executive organ.

It is not always easy to determine whether the patient has a loss or impairment in the structural relationships of inner speech, or in the attunement and adjustment between inner speech and the motor executive apparatus; the former is indicated when the patient himself is not clear on the position of the letters in the word.

The assumption of involvement of the motor executive organ in Ca (precentral gyrus) in anarthric and dysarthric complications appears to be proved by relevant anatomical findings (incapacity to produce sound, but soft whispering and definite impairment of the labials, is associated with lesion of the medulla); cases in which obscured previous dysarthric symptoms reappear during speech training after recovery from complete aphemia are similar, but are to be regarded as functional.

The fact that the corresponding organization of the articulatory factors is dependent on the ordered function of the assumed transmission mechanism makes it understandable that, apart from true dysarthria, similar disorders can occur through impairment of this mechanism (Liepmann speaks of "pseudo-dysarthric" disorders). As a rule, these cases show similar phenomena of the inner speech, viz. poor spelling and writing. Accordingly, for purely aphasic disorders and their anatomical substrates, any involvement (or localization) of the kinesthetic sensations and their schemata, assumed necessary for the regulation of the motor processes in the speech apparatus, is to be rejected as being of consequence only for the motor effect picture.

Against the interpretation of purely motor aphasic disorders as dysarthric (P. Marie), under various conditions (rote speaking, singing with lyrics, prefixing an automatized word to the otherwise impossible voluntary word) there is the completely correct articulation of words and sentences that otherwise cannot be produced or are produced poorly, and also the observation of occasional correct reading in the absence of spontaneous speech, and lastly, in polyglots, correct speech in one language with complete aphemia for another.

The symptoms of faciolingual apraxia are occasionally observed in the initial stage and usually disappear later. These seem to be juxtaposition effects on the corresponding (lowest) part of Ca and reflect the impossibility of voluntary initiation of the motor patterns in the executive apparatus and the consequent extension of the movements, rather like widespread associated movements appearing at the same time in the same area, as a sort of excess of effort.

The occasional disturbance of the intonation, more rarely defective accentuation, and the common monotony of utterance are all expressions of a disorder of the intonational pattern in the realm of phonology and indicate an involvement of the wider extent of Broca's area. The relative rarity of such disturbances is explained by the fact that intonation is a very early acquisition, preceding articulate speech and, therefore, is an especially automatized achievement. Moreover, since intonation stems from the emotional life, it is per se a more primitive feature.

Disturbances of the speech melody and especially of intonation may be due to the slowness and difficulty of speech in general, but when such disturbances extend into the period of speech recovery, we may assume that the musical elements of speech and especially the intonational structure have suffered.

H. Jackson has suggested the possibility that a number of the residual expressions (Help! God almighty!) may arise from emotional utterances ejaculated at the time of the stroke. It may be conjectured that the otherwise plastic anlage of the transmission mechanism has suddenly become rigid and reduced to a reflex-like response to a single expression. This lack of plasticity appears in the motor aphasic in the difficulty in abandoning an utterance once established. A somewhat similar phenomenon appears when an action or a sentence interrupted by a prolonged lapse of consciousness is then resumed where it left off.

We may also designate as secondary that part of the disturbance reflecting a loss of those factors which are due to practice. These become apparent here due to the great amount of practice involved in abbreviation and summarization which is characteristic of speech.

Accordingly, to mention only the most important features, we find the motor aphasic returning to previoiusly abandoned detours and indirect processes, with loss of automatization of numerous processes and the necessity of augmented effort for speech activation. This has the further consequence of increasing the awareness of the motor element, with a reduction in awareness for other functions. To the extent that normally the main part of the consciousness is directed toward the sense of the utterance, the mental formulation which precedes or accompanies speech is seriously impaired by this diversion of conscious activity. From this point of view, the motor aphasic might be compared to a pianist reduced to the state of a beginner, who (in accordance with the distinction between consciousness of content and consciousness of action) cannot (like the virtuoso—confident in the automatization of his motions) concentrate on the sense of the piece and the rendition of the most subtle interpretations, but must concentrate on the motor element, consciously thinking of every movement and motor component. This, of course, does not exclude the possibility that certain patterns of performance in the motor aphasic, such as the form of the sentence or the intonation, may be retained from the very beginning. To the defective distribution of conscious activity must be added the lowered capacity of our patients for the perception of words, which in turn seriously affects the content of what is to be said. If we further take into consideration that the span of consciousness is reduced, we begin to get an idea of the effect of this defect on the distribution of conscious activity. We are, finally, justified in assuming that all these factors adversely effect the spoken and mental formulation; for example, difficulty in finding words leading to the restructuring of the sentence and the search for periphrases.

Still other secondary disturbances of the intellectual component of speech are encountered, such as "losing the thread" of the discourse in consequence of failure of the sentence concept awaiting transmission through Broca's area. The essential disturbance here perhaps concerns the greater concentration on the motor aspect due to the speech difficulty. In a similar way the intention can also be disturbed in the presentation of the thought, the retention of content, and the direction of the thought. The extent to which such primary disturbances are involved (semiological or semantic disturbances) cannot be determined at this point, but they are suggested, for example, by the confusion of *yes* or *no* which occasionally extends well into the recovery period. This is not a result of incorrect transmission to the motor element, though of course a *lapsus linguae* and an inadequate attention to one's own utterance may be contributory factors. The phenomenon is sometimes too regular to dismiss the other assumption.

So-called motor agrammatism arising from the speech difficulties of the motor aphasic is also a secondary phenomenon. (For more on this subject, see p. 76).

Disturbances of speech frequently entail disorder of the various subfunctions brought together in the inner speech. Except in the early stages, this cannot be interpreted simply as a focal effect. Thus, in frontal aphasics there is at times a slight disturbance of comprehension for words and especially sentences. This may be due to general lowering of brain function, to poor retention of long speech formations, or as a result of inadequate psychic adjustment. Sound comprehension may be disturbed by loss of speech; occasionally, both in normals as well as word-deaf patients, articulation with the speaker is an aid to comprehension. Differences in linguistic type are probably important in the degree of the disturbances. The inability to retain long structures is a result of decreased activity and retention.

Articulation is usually detectable in reading with comprehension and in writing and may be prominent in speech disorders. It is observed when articulation is suppressed during reading or by the effect of linguistic errors and tends to regress with improvement in speech. In such cases, both linguistic skill and perhaps also the linguistic type are decisive.

Regarding the severe forms of *Horstummheit* (audimuditas), earlier designated as congenital aphasia, it later became clear, on the basis of other symptoms, that bilateral lesion of Broca's area was present (Pick, 1891). This was established as fact by Gianulli (1914). This is consistent with the fact that unilateral lesion of Broca's area in childhood, by virtue of the bilateral representation of speech at that age, does not lead to permanent motor aphasia. Apart from these organically determined forms, there are cases with defective development of acoustic responsiveness in the child. These can be eliminated or greatly improved with therapy.

The rare phenomena of *linguistic puerilism* and *modification of the character of the language* should be briefly mentioned. The former is a result of an acute lesion of the speech region. It has not yet been precisely discribed but is probably akin to total aphasia and to similar phenomena in senile atrophy. Agrammatism is a constant accompaniment and suggests a reversion to an infantile stage of development; a functional impairment in the speech organ is indicated by the phonetic change (economy of effort). Something similar is probably involved in the modification of the character of the language (in one of the rarest cases, agrammatism was also present), which is also due in part to phonetic change as well as changes in accentuation. These two phenomena are disturbances in the realm of phonology, their occurrence with aphasic disorders explained by the nearness of the pertinent cortical structures. The dialectal coloring of aphasic speech concerns the rule of Ribot.

The term *"temporal word deafness"* refers to rare cases of aphemia in connection with extensive unilateral lesion of the temporal lobe; in most cases, there are complications due to small foci in Broca's area, Insula, and internal capsule. There are also cases where extensive bilateral lesions of the temporal lobe, at times with involvement of occipital lobe, have resulted in a permanent defect of this type. That the absence of acoustic and optical excitation is the cause of this syndrome is refuted by cases of cortical deafness with retention of speech. The objection that "sound images" are lost with bilateral lesion in Wernicke's area is eliminated by the existence of different forms of central speech stimulation. Whatever the situation may be in a well-developed acoustic type, it concerns not just a speech disorder, but a psychic akinesia (Liepmann, 1908; Quensel, 1909; Henschen, 1920). This is supported by the striking contrast to the remainder of speech in cases of temporal lesions, as discussed below.

The function of Broca's area in pathology can be interpreted on the basis of its coordinative action, by which diverse stimuli are combined into ordered acts, leading to similarly ordered responses in the motor effector organ. This organ is compatible with the general principles formulated by Sherrington for central nervous system function.

According to Broca, the patient has lost *"le souvenir du proćedé, qu'il faut suivre pour articuler les mots,"* (the memory of the procedure that must be followed to articulate words). Certainly, some recovered patients report not knowing how individual letters or syllables were to be uttered. Such description is in keeping with what has been said regarding the opposition of *voluntary* and automatic initiation of the process, as a whole and in part, and to its disturbance in motor aphasia, without the necessity of accepting Broca's concept of a memory for the motor structures.

The question of the relationship between clinical severity and lesion extent, often obscured by the insoluble problem of neighboring effects, is frequently rendered superfluous by the fact that even a relatively small, appropriately placed lesion results in complete aphemia; one must also emphasize our lack of knowledge regarding the extent of any given "center."

Chapter 5

UNDERSTANDING OF SPEECH: THE PATH FROM SPEECH TO THOUGHT

An understanding of aphasic phenomena as disorders of the speech apparatus which conveys mental contents must be preceded by a full description and analysis of intact functions. This description is mainly psychological, due to our better knowledge of that aspect of the process. Based upon a clearly defined psychological localization, it is then possible to go beyond previous crude interpretations and strike out into the corresponding physiological processes *in cerebro*. While such considerations may at times be challenged by clinical discrepancies, this is of as little concern as the usual divergence between normal and pathological physiology. The error is sometimes on one side and sometimes on the other, but these differences can be resolved.

In the psychology of the speech function, there are two main fields to be considered: (1) that in which the mental content is converted into spoken expression, i.e. the path from thought to speech; and (2) the path from speech to thought, which represents that series of transitions between hearing and understanding.

With regard to the latter, the first prerequisite for the diagnosis of an aphasic disorder is adequate hearing. We must reject as inconclusive the assumption of a so-called speech scale (Sprachsext), according to which the undisturbed function of a specific range within a certain tuning-fork series is supposed to be a prerequisite for the differential diagnosis.

Our knowledge of the process of speech comprehension has advanced far beyond the older assumption of a two-stage subdivision (Wernicke's "primary identification"—recognition of the acoustic expression as such, "secondary identification"—understanding of that expression as a sign for a concept). However, we still know little about the various superimposed mechanisms and processes involved in speech comprehension and must be content with demonstrations, not always accepted, of levels of "contents" at particular stages. These may serve as guides to the understanding of these disorders in different stages of development, and these demonstrations, of course, frequently find their basis in pathology.

The basis of speech perception is in the serially ordered complexes of sound and noise sensation, which, modified by the speech melody, combine into "patterned" form. Initially in perception, the linguistic element becomes isolated from the diffuse total acoustic background. Then the word begins to differentiate, at first globally, on the basis of its recognition in memory as a phonetic unit, as an "auditory pattern" (Horgestalt). This generally obtains more readily for short words than for longer ones; then it is recognized as a component of language in general and then as belonging to a particular language. In the second phase, comprehension of the musical components of language takes place, i.e. the recognition of the language as belonging to a particular person, stemming perhaps from the "quality of familiarity." Similarities in auditory patterns may interfere with comprehension. The auditory patterns may, however, be perceived sufficient for general comprehension in spite of inadequate comprehension of individual phonemes. We know nothing about the individual processes concerned here and whether they actually correspond to different anatomical and physiological substrates (an arrangement in cortical layers, for example). Only the general lowering of function has been investigated experimentally, although other forms of dysfunction must certainly be considered.

In this stage, comprehension of the *sound of the word* is aided by an attuning of the executive speech apparatus to what is heard. This is a remnant of the infantile acoustic motor speech reflex, which with disinhibition may progress to repetition of what is heard with consequent improvement of the understanding. In correspondence with the phase of appreciation of the musical elements of speech, these too are occasionally repeated in isolation. Other sensory aids, e.g. objects, also help in sound comprehension. Moreover, the progressive understanding of the meaning of perceived words aids in the comprehension of subsequent word sounds. The situational background also has an effect, out of which develops the emotional and the objective, the significance of which in the analysis of perception is now generally accepted (Klemm, 1921).

The *understanding of words and sentences* is a more complicated process and is accomplished through a reactive emergence of the depths of memory. For this reason, it is less fully explained psychologically. This is especially so since the sentence, which seems to correspond to the ensemble of words heard in succession, is not merely the sum of the meaning of the individual words, but also contributes to the meaning of individual words. It was, therefore, erroneous to assume that this problem was explained by the assumption of a connection or assonance between the word and the concept or idea. Instead, this first takes place through the emergence of a general meaning-awareness (Messer's "sphere of awareness") which is then followed by the various complexes of symbols. A general awareness of direction, an intention, has a guiding effect. An inclination to assign a meaning, even to meaningless words, also plays a part. The words are thus objectively determined; concepts or parts of concepts may also be vehicles of meaning or may only be manifestations of the understanding. Then comes the conception of word categories and of the grammatical form of the word. With the understanding of the first words heard, sentence comprehension begins through a kind of preconstruction (K. Buhler), aided by the fact that two successive words are involuntarily brought into relationship through a tendency to form combinations. This is built up on the intonational pattern which develops from the musical components heard and on the derived syntactical model. The latter plays a part in the differentiation of words into names for things and for actions, as vehicles of sentence meaning, which suffice for the understanding of simple sentences. In such a case, words expressing relationships (prepositions, adverbs, conjunctions) may not be noted, as they are less essential. Ordinarily a content pattern is developed in the listener by way of the frequent experience of analogy formation, which corresponds to the expressive thought pattern of the speaker. It is achieved through successive meanings applied to words, whose occasional ambiguity is compensated for by the meaning of the sentence. The development of the thought in the listener may either take place by the completion of the syntactical pattern by the thing described, or the thing described may serve to clarify the content (Bühler, 1923), or there may be a mixture of the two. That which is spoken and the thought or thought-complex which it generates are thus gradually fitted into the mental situation common to listener and speaker. This is a *gestalt* factor that plays a great part in determining comprehension, with mimicry and gesture playing an important supporting role (as when pointing replaces a part of the sentence).

In the understanding of complex sentences, the intermediate-experience-relationships, (*Zwischenerlebnisbeziehungen*) of Bühler play an important role (concerning the path from thought to speech) by insuring the unity of the awareness-content as expressed in the parts (the "thread" of the discourse), demanding, of course, retention of the preceding events.

This description of stages in the realization of speech comprehension should be qualified by the fact that even in the normal case these stages do not occur one right after the other, but rather limit each other (word comprehension begins with the first words heard), so that word meaning may be grasped even before the sound of the words has been completely taken in, or sentence meaning before the meaning of the individual words. The process will also be variously compressed according to whether the utterance is to serve as an announcement, a statement, or a description. The first two instances concern mainly an emotionally directed form, the feeling for which, based on the musical elements of language, facilitates and demarcates the process; in this instance, as well as others, less important words are hardly taken into account. The process is also abbreviated by the commonly used expressions and phrases which characterize ordinary discourse. Lastly, to this entire account of the processes of word and sentence comprehension, it should be added that other processes certainly play a part which, not being conscious, cannot be dealt with at this time.

Chapter 6

THE PATH FROM THOUGHT TO SPEECH

CONSIDERATION OF THE path from thought to speech reveals a number of stages in which the thought processes, with increasing intensity, converge along a common path to the motor executive organ. If the number of stages in the total process appears greater than on the impressive side, this is due to the fact that the psychological analysis of expressive speech is further advanced and also to the greater variety of relevant data in the pathological symptoms. As the very formulation of the question shows, we proceed on the assumption, now widely accepted, that thinking and speaking are not identical or even parallel, though they often run together in close relationship.

The steps constituting the path from thought to speech, though not precisely understood, may yet be classified in two groups: that of *thought formulation* and that of *linguistic formulation*. As in the case of the impressive process, their sequence is generally incomplete and will not always run in a prescribed order. However, as previously discussed, depending on the purpose of speech and the underlying emotional factors, which in turn directly induce habitual syntactical and grammatical constructions, there is sometimes, even in an early stage, a fragmentary linguistic formulation as a kind of "manifestation" or "release" (Bühler). But, even in formulation as "statement" or "description," there is often a displacement of the processes of linguistic and thought formulation with respect to each other.

Often, thought is linguistically formulated at its very inception, just as everyday speech makes use of ready-made sequences of words, cliches, and sentences. Even here, there is a definite relationship between thought and speech, although in a much shortened and more automatized form. The more one thinks in words, the greater the possibility that true aphasic disturbances, at the boundary between intuitive and discursive thinking, shift closer toward thinking than is otherwise the case.

Finally, an especially important feature is that not everything which is conceived and meant to be aroused in the thought of the listener is linguistically expressed in ordinary communication. There is instead a spoken stenogram, supplemented to an important extent by the objective and subjective *situation* through *mimicry* and *gesture*. This is especially important in appraising differences in communication, since the factors mentioned afford the greatest economy of both mental and linguistic performance. The intellectual formulation of thought, which often presents initially in an undifferentiated fashion, develops gradually, but assumes an increasing clarification based upon that part of awareness with which it develops. This is derived from experience and knowledge which is ordered, with due regard for object relations as well as the subjective relationships grounded in the speaker between these components, into a sequence of topics, a sort of thought pattern. This preparation for a predicative arrangement takes place either by analytic reduction of actions or objects or by the synthesis of the component parts.

On the basis of this structuring of the thought, the *second step* is now taken. The linguistic formulation will develop during the stage of mental analysis as a successive formulation or, after that analysis, as a subsequent formulation based upon the various *linguistic means* unique to that language, such as tone, accentuation, tempo, word order, and grammatization. The order of appearance depends on whether an exclamation, a command, or a statement is involved. First an *accentuation pattern* (Betonungsschema) and then a *sentence patten* (Satzschema) develop, which concern in their formation the topical sequence arising from the *thought pattern* (Gedankenschema) and the feeling-tone derived from that order. In other words, the feeling for the word order (syntax) and the linguistic feeling (Sprachgefühl), developed before formal schooling, initially play an important role. In comparison, the grammatical rules acquired later recede into the background in ordinary speech, especially since the application of any rule interferes with the fine adjustment of the linguistic formulation to thought.

With regard to the accentuation pattern, this is not a single entity, as is seen by the various accents and their independent loss, but is rather the sum of several processes.

Following this, the usually automatic process of *word finding* and the arrangement of the words in the sentence pattern takes place. First appear the meaning-laden words which correspond to objects (and actions) in the thought pattern. This is a complicated process, since the sentence meaning is expressed only through the meanings that result from the mutual influences in the lexical entry process. This is then followed by the insertion of the grammatical words and then, as an expression of the syntactical interrelationships, by the *grammatization* of the content words. Also occurring in this process, in an analogous way, are the feeling-tones mentioned above.

In protracted speech, Bühler's (1908) "intermediate-experience-relationships" come into consideration. This concerns relationships between thoughts, between the thought and the immediate task, as well as other current tasks, and relationships of the speaker to the content. If these are lacking, especially the initial group, there is a loss in unity and control; the "thread" of the conversation is easily lost.

Then, on the basis of structural groupings which correspond to the inner-speech organization, successive activation of correlated processes in the speech executive organ takes place. Similarly, the transmission-mechanism discussed with the development of speech comes into play.

The assumption of the conductance to the motor executive apparatus of more or less fixed engrams appears to be negated by the coming into play of parts of the intonational pattern during the process, in addition to other arguments showing the word to be a dynamic formation. In order to understand the functions involved in this transmission and their disorders, it must be emphasized that prior to the actual transmission, the complex thought content is virtually present in an abbreviated and condensed form. Through successive differentiation (analysis) the sequential excitation of the corresponding structures comes about via more or less automatized speech impulses.

We have discussed the leading role of the sound pictures in the initial development of speech. In the increasing automatization of this excitation which leads to speech, the sound picture soon becomes superfluous. However, should difficulties occur, even in normals, it may reassert itself (as will be discussed later from psychological experimentation, regarding the elimination of circumlocutions and the deletion of component actions with increasing practice and skill).

We may regard as the nodal point of the common paths involved in the transmission process the area first indicated by Broca and situated in the posterior portion of the first frontal convolution (on the left side) without being able to specify more precisely the extent of the area involved. The magnitude and the refinement of the functions in question account for the size of this central area. The area is anatomically predetermined and is dominant over the motor executive organ localized in the lower part of Ca.

We can best understand the disturbances of the transmission process by observations on typing and telegraphy. With increasing automatization, a hierarchy of habitual patterns is formed which clearly corresponds to the sequence of stages of the described processes.

Looked at from a more general point of view, the two mechanisms centered in Broca's and Wernicke's areas represent a higher type of transformer and reducer, such as used to describe telephone equipment.

Chapter 7

INNER SPEECH, THE TRANSMISSION MECHANISM AND THEIR ANATOMICAL LOCALIZATION

CENTRAL TO THE transmission process sketched here is what is better designated as the "inner word" (corresponding to the prime element of the sentence) than as "inner speech." This represents a synthesis of mechanisms, beginning with the acoustic motor reflex system described above in connection with the development of speech, which has come into existence in the following way. Words conceived, heard and later read will together form perceptual structures and will give rise to motor phonetic patterns. These develop into tightly organized response relationships which react as a whole even though only a component is activated. Since it is first to develop, the acoustic component is generally the first to be aroused. Stimulation in thinking, reading and writing leads automatically to activation of the speech units in the motor effector organ. This interrelatedness explains the clinically important fact that anatomical or functional disorders at any point in the speech field will impair the inner speech wholly or in part, including its functional participation in more distantly localized mechanisms. It is not very likely that the differentiation of second hand speech (written language) will have a major disturbing influence upon the older sound-picture. This relationship accounts for the fact, which is important from the standpoint of therapy, that when some component of this normally interwoven complex fails, another immediately and automatically substitutes. Even in normals, under various conditions, different components may play a decisive role; predisposition (type of thought and of language), the level of intellectual development, the nature of the acquisition, later practice in the various components and even chance. These facts are of clinical significance in each individual case. Accordingly, it is not valid to construct a specific schema of the speech process, which is identical for all individuals, from the standpoint of the acoustic part of inner speech. We may regard as inner speech, the form of excitation of the motor speech apparatus that has become habitual for that individual; ordinarily, as we have said, this is the acoustic motor form. A motor form has been described in cases where the reflex excitation of motor impulses intrudes, in an especially intense manner, into the consciousness of the individual in question, such that it is felt as a tendency to motion or as actual motion.

This transmission is monitored from two separate directions: first, the motor effects of the excitation are adjusted to the thought form and content (especially with respect to the musical elements of language), the higher psychic processes being decisive; second, these processes exert a regulating effect and thereby prevent an impairment due to the automatization of such processes as those of thought, but also of writing.

Both of these regulative controls involve the centers regarded as transmission sites to the expressive functions (for speech, Broca's area in F3; for writing, the foot of F2). It is thus understandable that interruption of transmission by lesion of these centers inactivates the regulations, the transmission obscuring their function.

While this is all we know concerning the first group of controls with respect to the second group, we are much better informed through psychological studies by American authors of typing and telegraphy. A summary of these investigations (Lewin, 1922) discloses the following factors found in an analysis of practice effects to contribute to the acceleration of performance (Book, 1908). These include elimination of detours and side processes, shifts in the sequence of processes, reduction of the degree of awareness with increasing automatization, fusion of several acts into a whole activated by a single volitional impulse (sentence and sentence groups), and earlier setting of activation stimuli.

With the refined development of writing as an expression of thoughts, a center analogous to Broca's center has developed in that part of F2 situated anterior to the relevant motor centers. What has been said of Broca's center for speech is also true of the writing center.

All of the objections that have been raised, obviously not without justification, against this "writing" center (improperly so designated) are refuted by this interpretation of the psychic regulations (because of the possibility of writing with the head, the legs, it was alleged necessary to assume a special center for each activity). Centers similar to those for expression are also found on the receptive side. That for auditory comprehension has been discussed. A similar one has developed in the region of the angular gyrus, where graphic symbols are perceived as a special kind of optical impression and then conveyed to the intellect as symbols for thoughts. For obvious reasons, we are less informed about processes in the receptive centers than those on the expressive side. Volition is much more important in the latter, and is of clinical significance in that the receptive functions, being similar, are more easily restored.

In closing, mention should be made here of the method, reported by Proust-Lichtheim-Dejerine, of determining the condition of inner speech through reports by motor aphasics of letters or syllables in otherwise unpronounceable words. Apart from difficulties intrinsic to the disease itself, this wholly artificial test is unsatisfactory for the reason that it is derived from the written form and incorrectly assumes that letters and phonemes, syllables and speech groups coincide. This division is untenable even linguistically (there are not isolated sound images). It is a process acquired in late school years and is commonly not retained long. It does not take account of the silent letters, and it is obvious that in such a matter we must consider the extent to which the "gestalt" of the whole word was a decisive factor in learning to read. Of relevance with regard to this and other ingenious methods of investigation are the findings of psychological experimentation (Lewin, cited on page 36) based on the concept of structure and *gestalt*, as to the incapacity for a component action which has been learned as a part of another action. An attempt to apply similar methods to the analogous field of apraxia would suffice to make clear their untenability.

Chapter 8

DOMINANCE OF THE LEFT HEMISPHERE, SIGNIFICANCE OF THE RIGHT

U<small>P TO THIS POINT</small> we have been discussing the speech apparatus as a unit without regard to the anatomicophysiological fact of the paired nature of the cerebrum. We shall now consider the fact, which is valid for all forms of aphasia, that in right-handed individuals, it is usually lesions of the left hemisphere which lead to aphasic disorders, while in similar lesions on the right side aphasia is either absent or minimal.

With regard to the cause and nature of this left hemispheric preference, we may say the following: it coincides with human right-handedness, about 90 percent; this along with left-hemispheric dominance is due mainly to an inherited physio-anatomical superior development of the right hand. In individual and social development (emotion, speech, gesture) this leads to greater use of that hand with the consequence that the more advanced and presumably superior development of the left cerebral hemisphere probably plays the decisive role. This may be related to the law of economy which is operative even in normals (e.g. influence of situational factors on the extent of that which is to be expressed in speech), in that the "higher" intellectual functions as "patterned" entities, which are interposed between the end points of the receptor and executive organs, as in the transmission of the physical correlates of thoughts through Broca's area to the motoric center, are completely lacking in lateralized characteristics and are therefore inaccessible to such a division.

In spite of the relatively symmetrical location of the cortical regions associated with higher psychic functions in the two hemispheres, their combined work should not be interpreted as bilateral in the same sense as in the expressive and receptive organs which are bilaterally present and function symmetrically. There are no left-side or right-side thoughts (or parts of thoughts), and accordingly their linguistic expression and their development from the bilateral acoustic receptive organs can occur only through a single transmission organ (simple reflection shows the similarity of this line of thought to cases of agnosia and apraxia, insofar as the latter are direct expressions of the psychic). Incidentally, this eliminates difficulties regarding the extent to which the executive organs may work together symmetrically in the adult.

It is only when we keep this in mind that the primacy of the sentence as the unit of thought acquires its deeper justification.

The priority of one hemisphere must therefore develop and will be less apparent in the lower functions (see the instrumental disorders in amusia). This is also *furthered* by writing with the right hand, as a conversion of mental entities into motor acts.

The behavior of left-handed individuals is opposite to that described for dextrals. However, there are a few poorly explained cases which, in spite of right-handedness, have right-sided lesions followed by aphasic defects. Lastly, a few cases have been reported in which the pertinent foci are partly in one and partly in the other hemisphere. This phenomenon, probably related to ambidexterity, is explained by the conflict of a predisposition (e.g. to right-brainedness) with individual (latent) left-brainedness. It may also be possible that dominance may undergo a change, as under the influence of education in writing; however, illiterates also show preponderance of the left hemisphere. The fact that the left hemisphere is frequently dominant does not exclude the participation of the right hemisphere in these processes, even for adults. On the contrary, such participation is demonstrated by the finding that even in right-handed individuals, right-sided lesions, especially in the region of the speech executive organs, are followed by the same phenomena, though of briefer duration (of course, the possibility of diaschisis in such cases remains open). However, the participation of the right hemisphere alone does not ordinarily suffice to maintain speech function.

In childhood the two hemispheres normally work together, inevitably due to the bilateral arrangement of the pertinent acoustic organs. It is believed that the usual rapid compensation of childhood aphasia can be explained on this basis, but fixed aphasias have also been observed in children after unilateral lesions. It is only later, with the development of the intellectual organs to which the receptive and executive speech organs are subordinate, that the initiative priority of the left hemisphere develops. This is in accordance with what has been said regarding the unitary nature of intellect (similarly, one occasionally notes a unilateral basis for pseudobulbar paralysis). The speech fields are trained on both sides, but transmission into the expressive and resolution out of the impressive take place only on one side. Apart from their evident practical (surgical) importance, these theoretical problems are closely connected with the question of substitute functions, to which we shall return later.

Chapter 9

GENERAL POINTS OF VIEW TO BE TAKEN INTO CONSIDERATION IN THE INTERPRETATION OF PATHOLOGICAL PHENOMENA

THE DESCRIPTION OF aphasic disorders and attempts at their interpretation must now be prefaced by a few further observations of general significance. Since it is not yet possible to explain aphasic disorders on the basis of pathological changes, we must rely upon a systematic presentation of the pertinent factors and their nature. As in the natural sciences, the *developmental idea* is the guiding principal; we speak of *degeneration of cerebral functions* which, as in the course of recovery, has an analogous role in their development. But a distinction must be made between true degeneration (for example, in simple atrophy) and focal disorders which destroy structure and function in an irregular manner. Similarly, their recovery in the adult brain differs from their development in the child. Only in functional cases does the recovery from a disorder which affects a single organ take place, perhaps quite analogous to the original stages of development.

"*Ribot's rule*" represents the direct expression of the developmental idea. Thus, in the speech field as a whole as well as within its component parts, the oldest functions offer the greatest resistance to slow degeneration, while the youngest are the first to be involved (in acute, indiscriminately destructive lesions, of course, the rule does not hold or at best is only valid for their chronic aftereffects). Occasionally on an accidental basis, the greater automatization of later-acquired functions provides an exception to the rule and shows that it is not age in itself, but rather its resultant degree of automatization that determines the increased resistance.

Regarding the organic substrate, we suggest that the improved readiness to respond is due to *practice,* the integrated organization of nervous elements, and perhaps also to the effects of practice on structural growth, as assumed by some (Vernon, 1907; Collier, 1920, 1921).

With respect to loss of certain categories of words, observations that persist in the literature as examples of Ribot's rule may be criticized as irrelevant and in urgent need of review, since they are taken from case histories with no regard to functional differences.

We distinguish on the basis of causation *organic* and *functional* disorders, but it must be noted that even organic disorders are not limited to the immediate effects of the lesion, but also result in wider disorders of a functional nature (see especially von Monakow's theory of diaschisis).

In accordance with the theory, empirically confirmed, that every organic disorder corresponds to a similar one of functional determination, we should consider here those functional aphasic disorders which are of a transitory nature. They are provoked by gout, Bright's disease, uremia, diabetes, sunstroke, migraine, toxic (tobacco) and infectious factors, arteriosclerosis and arteriospasm, mental exhaustion, epileptic, eclamptic, and paralytic attacks. Lastly, in the early stage of organic lesions (brain tumor, vascular changes) similar transitory phenomena are found which are nonetheless functional. Conversely, the functional nature of some of the complaints mentioned is doubtful. In both categories there is a similarity of form according to which the pathological phenomena divide into defects and qualitative functional disturbances. Their interpretation is as complicated as their observation appears simple. The immediate and poorly known disruptive factors affect their appearance and also the many restitutional processes interact, along with the whole brain and the speech apparatus, with the lesion and its functional effects. But there is also a third factor in the development of the symptoms. We now know that positive symptoms may be due to defects, and that primitive processes, ordinarily inhibited by or associated with superordinate functions, can be released by defect or absence of inhibiting functions, i.e. by *disinhibition* with resultant modification of the clinical picture. It is known from psychological experimentation that the "task" has an inhibiting effect on secondary activities.

The significance of disinhibition is not yet well known. It appears in the primitive form of release phenomena, as well as in cases where the patients themselves admit to such involuntary processes. While in some cases the coherence of an associated function normally prevents the occurrence of another, more frequently the absence or reduction in control by a higher function disinhibits a subordinate function (see the discussion below concerning logorrhea and paraphasia). The precise circumstances for the duration of the disinhibition are still unknown; it can only be said that the restoration of the inhibiting processes plays a decisive role. In contrast to these crude release phenomena, it is not known to what extent disinhibitions are also involved within the component parts of functional relationships. However, in accordance with what is known from the general physiology of the central nervous system, we shall always have to consider, in our attempts at explanation, the ubiquitous *interplay of stimulation and inhibition.*

Unquestionably, on the *impressive* side of speech, there are similar pathological disinhibitions. If they are absent, it must be due to the nature of these speech processes, which are almost entirely removed from volitional and conscious control.

There occurs a similar phenomenon, analogous to the effects of lesion of the superior colliculus (Head), in occasional cases of acoustic hyperesthesia, along with acoustic unresponsiveness in patients with word deafness.

Another and no less important aspect must be recognized in the *opposition between volition and automatism,* common in pathological states and also here in view of the extreme automatization of speech processes. Generally we can say that even in the development of speech as a child, the automatic component necessary for the voluntary induction and maintenance of speech may be impeded or made impossible, and that any such impedence of an otherwise subconscious act it registered as a conscious difficulty. We have made reference earlier to the various facts derived from the realm of psychological experiment regarding the "practice" factor and which may be relevant for evaluation of disrupted automatism.

In certain cases of aphasia, comparison of the modes of action with those of the normal individual reveals obvious regression to a stage of minimal or nonexistent training, which does not need further mention. The one point we wish to make is that the associated movements which accompany the recovery from aphemia and thereafter decline indicate that loss of automatism entails also loss of the motor and regulatory actions which lead to that automatism. Thus, there is a defect of the preparatory stages of motion and these (see page 15) become shifted into the foreground of motor aphasia. Also belonging here and necessitated by the disorder is the construction of extensive control processes which only gradually disappear again and which greatly impede the mechanization of the whole.

The general factors will also be frequently mentioned in the discussion of specific instances. Let us mention here that in the regression of the voluntary into the automatic, the advantage of relying on the automatic can be clearly observed clinically.

On the impressive side, as mentioned above, volition plays a less evident part, and in accordance with this no conclusions can be drawn from its opposition to automatism. Nonetheless, we can say that the contrast brought out by the lesion between the severe loss of automatism and its incipient restoration is of significance, and this obtains even more for the control functions.

This discussion of symptoms and the recognition of general factors important for their interpretation would be incomplete if we made no further note of the various *reparatory processes*. In nonprogressive cases, these begin more clearly, and usually acutely after the shock effects of the focal disorder have diminished, and modify the picture in complex and varied ways. They are divided into *genuine reparatory* processes, depending on the nature of the lesion (functional or gross anatomical) and a purely functional *restitution* which may be mixed with organic restitution, which concerns regions affected directly and those affected indirectly through sympathy. Secondarily, there are *substitutions* (compensations) either by immediately adjacent regions or by areas functionally related to the region damaged (see comments regarding "makeshifts" in reference to inner speech). There is compensation also by the homologous part of the opposite hemisphere which has the same structure as and is in functional relationship with the affected area (so that here also there is sometimes restitution). The multiplicity of these factors, along with what has been said of the disruptive factors, gives us an indication of the difficulties, indeed of the impossibility, of establishing their precise role in any individual case. In fact, even the most exacting autopsy findings do not resolve all doubts, since they provide but uncertain answers to questions of function. All that can be done here is to define the general aspects.

In the rebuilding of the damaged area, it is chiefly the anatomical factors that are to be considered. Regarding the repair of adjacent regions, it is established that only those areas of similar structure will be capable of similar function. When this is not the case, and it is usually not because of the small size of the homogeneous cortical areas, we shall be dealing not with true restitution but with functional substitution via "detours" (compensation) by "makeshifts," as in the cooperation of areas functionally related to that under stress. On casual inspection, this compensation may be quite similar to the intact function, but upon closer inspection, particularly with regard to its production, the circuitous route will be evident and will make the resultant function understandable. The possibility and onset of such compensations are determined by both distant and neighboring effects, and their appraisal is hindered by the fact that such effects may extend in the direction of the other hemisphere as well.

With respect to those compensations achieved by circuitous routes, the normal participation in the speech function of the "other" hemisphere, ordinarily the right one, is the primary determining factor. It is generally true that the receptor functions, especially auditory comprehension, which have a greater degree of bilateral representation and are also free of the complicating factor of volition, show a more rapid recovery from these disorders.

In general, the more rapid recovery, *ceteris paribus,* is taken as a criterion for the participation of the other hemisphere. However, we must take into consideration, more than previously, what has been said concerning the rapid and automatic involvement of makeshifts by the functionally related regions. In any case, the principal determining factor will be the qualitative aspect of the performance, the temporal factor will be considered only when demonstrable hereditary influences are involved, e.g. hereditary left-handedness, hemiplegia of the right side (of the brain) with aphasia, rapid recovery from the latter (as a possible manifestation of the normal partial participation of *both* Broca's regions in speech).

Lastly, we should emphasize that one functional disorder may be *overlaid* by another, such that the first cannot come to light until the one which overlies it has receded. Thus, a severe functional disturbance naturally conceals a similar and less severe one, e.g. agraphia conceals a disorder of the orthography, which appears when the agraphia resolves. Even a serious defect can also be concealed at first by a separate disorder; a frontal aphemia may conceal a temporal echolalia or paraphasia, which are not apparent until the former is resolved. The distinction between such phenomena and those having to do with recovery is clear without further comment.

As has been mentioned, an important role is played in scientific understanding by the effects *in the vicinity and at a distance* that accompany all focal disorders, especially those of acute onset. To these more or less diffusely distributed factors, von Monakow (in his theory of diaschisis) has added still others: elective, anatomically oriented, organically and functionally effective. These are of greater significance here than in general brain pathology, for not only greatly refined mechanisms but also mechanisms appearing externally by their functions are involved. Their interpretation as inhibitory has been contested because of the impossibility of determining their chronological effects, but many facts of speech pathology nevertheless justify this interpretation.

Of course, this situation and the reparatory processes related to its disappearance are both quantitatively and qualitatively *dependent on the general condition of the particular brain in question*. In order to clarify this, we may point out the contrast between the youthful or still vigorous normal organ and its capacity for complete functional recovery in spite of a permanent focal defect and the senescent brain, which is not only less likely to compensate but also more easily exhausted. Not only the condition of the brain but also the general state of health will be of importance in this regard. This can be clearly seen from the reports of master typists that the slightest change in the general state of health has a marked effect on performance. This leads directly to the factor of *fatigue,* which is manifest both generally and in specific organs.

Let us preface the following discussion of *psychic factors* with the remark that these are also paralleled by physical factors, and that only our deficient knowledge of this aspect justifies the formal dichotomy.

Here belongs the fact that the *reduced level of awareness* in the aphasic is greater than in other cerebral disorders. Clearly, all the functions which serve to combine certain arrangements and details into a single entity are particularly affected. The important factor of proper *distribution of attention,* often noted by the patient himself as defective, is dependent on this and on the narrowed range of awareness. The varying difficulty of processes and the consequent direction of attention to them has a particularly disturbing effect. Not only are the automatization of habits of use which accompany the lowered awareness affected but also concomitant modes of control and/or new acquisition of behavior patterns which are based primarily on an economical distribution of the attention. The demonstration of this defect leads to other observations. First, in every utterance a distinction may be made between the sounds pronounced, their meaning, and the basic underlying content, so that any disturbance of the proper distribution of attention among the three may severely damage the result. The very multiplicity of these factors has a further effect toward increasing the difficulty; also, the chronological relationship between thinking and speaking, with the initiative taken by the thought, and finally the intensification of every disturbance by the direction of attention toward the act in question, which itself may not be seriously disordered. This fact, which can be proved for the executive side, can be assumed to hold also for the impressive side.

The importance of the lowered *perceptiveness* and *memory* must be mentioned here. The fact that these can be disordered in varying degrees for the different speech components accounts for the variety of such effects. However, in this respect we have not advanced much beyond general observations and do not, for instance, know to what extent differences between mechanical and logical memory obtain.

In order to avoid misunderstandings let us also emphasize that the factors of attention, limits of awareness, and so on can be discussed only in respect of their effects, since only by a precise clinical differentiation of nonaphasic factors will it be possible to determine the aphasic factors.

We should mention another generally observed factor, one that occupies a central position between the psychic and the somatic. Particularly with regard to expression processes, we shall frequently be able to demonstrate a law of *economy*. Though it is more clearly manifest here, it is also encountered on the impressive side. (In precaution, let us emphasize that we are not dealing here with a conscious effect; let us also note its presence in the performance of early childhood).

In this regard, we should again mention the importance of the *external situation,* which is objectively and subjectively determined according to what is common to speaker and hearer, tester and testee. Even in ordinary communication this factor often leads to a marked but unnoticed simplification of speech. (Also note its beneficial effect on otherwise frequently ambiguous terms.) This explains the difference between the patient's behavior at home and in the laboratory; it also refers to the influence of the milieu, which in turn determines the *inner situation,* again with the resultant salutory effect of successful function on the patient himself.

We should also mention here the "attunement," a term applied by von Kries to certain processes not detectable in awareness which modify or facilitate the connections or the occurrence of other cerebral processes (connective or dispositional tuning; as an example of the norm, see the effect of the musical key). One is tempted to explain the role of dispositional attunement in attention on the basis of the demonstrated centrifugal fibers shown to exist in the sensory paths. This mechanism also applies for the interpretation of certain phenomena occurring in word deafness (for example, the question of sensory responsiveness). Even in regions corresponding to the higher psychic processes, similar though shorter centrifugal paths probably exist which serve for such adjustments (attunement to different languages, to different word spheres, and different lines of thought). The importance of the situation as a factor in attunement is evident without further discussion, and probably "makeshifts" can be regarded from this point of view.

Further, the contrast between automatism and volition also comes into play. Attunement is a process which is predominantly automatic and unconscious and can be replaced by an act of volition only with difficulty and inadequately if at all.

Regarding a factor that may be disruptive in the recovery stage of lesions, we should also remember the difficulty, known from normals as well, of eliminating "bad" structures established by habit, not only motor structures, in favor of better ones. It is evident that this is important in attempts to cure by exercise, for only through exercise are the "good" structures regained.

Lastly, we should note the considerable *variation in the intensity of the disorders,* which may result either from the general state of the brain or from obscure factors affecting the areas under stress or even from the less clear psychic factors; some of these have been mentioned. It is evident in view of the multitude of proven disruptive factors which are involved that individual cases can be explained in only the most general terms, and that we will often have to be satisfied with confusions based on the normal with determining as nearly as possible the functional areas involved.

A word remains to be said about *patient's self-observation,* which when obtained from persons of a high intellectual level can certainly be very instructive (and even those of less intelligent patients can be enlightening), but which must be subjected in every case to a criticism based on theory. We know from psychological experimentation that even when normal experimental subjects have performed incorrectly, they believe themselves to have performed correctly. With the aid of such observations we can better appraise the significance of *imaginal and speech types* as expressions of individual variation. The influence of these variations can no longer be denied; in general the customary type related to specific functions does not become clearly evident until difficulties in performing those functions arise. The significance of the various types will, of course, appear in different ways according to the nature of the disordered function in question. Disorders of the optic-imaginal type would be of particular importance in the relation to semiology where descriptions are concerned (cf. the importance of visual images for the style of young people) (Kroh, 1922) or in connection with the disturbance of orientation first described by Förster.

Attempts have been made to correlate the cortical histology of certain areas with the physiological functions attributed to them and to exploit this relationship in the interpretation of pathological phenomena, e.g. with respect to the acoustic center. However, these constructions do not parallel the clinically better known regions (visual cortex), and for that reason their application to pathology seems out of the question for now. The same is true of the various interpretations, based on histological structure of processes related to neural elements in a general way, which have not yet advanced beyond the realm of the speculative. With regard to the idea of mutual adjustment and compensation of the neuron systems in question, we should mention a suggestion of Piéron (1921) for evaluating Lapicque's theory of chronaxie. Henschen (1920-1922) also set up a working hypothesis analogous to wireless telegraphy (Jolly had already suggested something of the kind). It remains quite unclear how this can be brought into harmony with the often postulated paths connecting the centers.

Recently an attempt has been made to go beyond the pathophysiological and resort to physical concepts (Pötzl, 1923), such as energy and its various forms, for the interpretation of certain phenomena. Apart from the complicating multiplicity of factors involved in the individual case (Eliasberg, 1923), there are two reasons for special caution: first, our little knowledge of the relation between physiological and physical processes; and second, the fact that precisely those actions which are accomplished promptly are automatized and so take place with a minimum of energy. Moreover, the same or similar actions can be induced in psychologically different ways so that conclusions regarding the energy consumed become very precarious. Accordingly, occasional attempts to treat the performance of patients numerically have led to widely fluctuating results, in which the influence of the discussed somatic factors play an important role. All that can be said with certainty in pathology is that every plus in function at one place simultaneously damages or impedes ongoing functions in other places. Empirical estimates on the basis of the symtoms alone as to the difficulty of this or that component process are therefore entirely justified.

These attempts to grasp at least the nature of the processes are hindered by the complexity and obscurity of the symptoms. Only the clinicopsychological study of the details of the relationships, which has surpassed the analysis now begun of the gross symptoms of aphemia, alexia, and so on, can prepare the way for anatomicophysiological understanding.

A few words must be devoted to the *close association of motor aphasic and agraphic disorders with apraxia,* as discussed especially by Liepmann (1913), although no direct use will be made of these theories. Even if we should concede with great reservation the essential similarity in the two sets of symptoms, conditions are such that the aphasic phenomena, in spite of their complexity, are much clearer, even genetically, so as to better clarify the apraxic phenomena than vice versa. Our reservation concerns the divergence of "purposes": in speaking, the sense of what is to be said is the sole purpose; the resultant effect does not lie in the sounds produced, but in their psychological effect. In actions, this is true only in those cases which come under the heading of sign language. Moreover, there is no reason to entertain the notion of a movement plan, especially in speaking, even if we were to admit such a thing in general. According to our discussion of the development of speech and our arguments therefrom, the notion of an "acoustic" plan is no less likely, and its rejection is fully justified by the fundamental importance of the sentence.

Accordingly, a clarification of aphasic phenomena by means of interpretations developed in apraxia theory seems rather unpromising. This of course is not meant to deny the kinship of the two series of phenomena, as in the common factors of causation, and in consequence the frequent parallels between the two.

Thus, to mention only one matter, there can hardly be any doubt that the concepts of Gestalten, structures, and so on used here can be applied directly to the theory of apraxia. However, only by reworking these concepts from the above point of view and with regard to voluntary action can we hope to relate the two fields in a systematic fashion. Similar relationships apply to the different forms of agnosia; there can be no doubt as to the similarity, in principle, of word-deafness and word-blindness to the types of agnosia here discussed, since both involve processing at different levels of observation in respect to psychic activity. But we still have insufficient knowledge of these relationships to offer a systematic explanation. Those transfers that are possible, especially in the acoustic sphere, are similarly acknowledged.

In this regard, a further consideration should be noted, as a guide for future discussion and to bring the functional, dynamic discussion of phenomena into harmony with patho-anatomical findings. This should prove better than the focal interpretations which have been the rule up to now.

It has generally been observed, especially for the temporal lobes with their multitude of individual phenomena within a relatively small area, that both small and larger foci of apparently equal extent, confirmed on serial section, often differ strikingly in symptomatology. Such differences are naturally all the more striking when, after the subsidance of functional conditions (diaschisis), they not only remain but sometimes appear more strongly.

For an understanding of this phenomenon, we may resort to the *difference between focal and functional arrangement of the centers in question,* now clearly evident in the regions of cortical, sensory and visual localization. While this has not been demonstrated for other functional areas, especially higher ones close to the intellectual, it probably exists for these as well.

However, these facts show that the higher the functional position of the organ or part of an organ in question, the more its functional organization predominates and develops. We are therefore probably justified in assuming a highly developed functional localization for the temporal lobes as a part of the speech field. This does not account for the difficulty of symptom variation with the same focus, since if the localization were fixed, the neuron groups corresponding to the same functional relationships would also correspond to the same focus. This difficulty is eliminated by the fact that the function creates its own neuron groups, both quantitatively and qualitatively different, as in normals, according to the nature of its development. When we consider this as well as individual factors, the differences in relation to the same focus become understandable. Moreover, it is clear that functional localization is a result of the "Gestalts" and "structures."

It cannot be our task to extend this reasoning to the various fields; we wish only to point out that it also applies to the interpretation of the different symptom pictures of motor aphasia. It is also evident that this interpretation permits a more precise formulation to the question of the extent to which the "whole" cortex or only a part is used in the processes of higher psychic function.

Chapter 10

PARAPHASIA

THE DESCRIPTION and interpretation of *temporally conditioned speech disorders* should again be prefaced with the statement that although the temporal part of the speech field is considered as the sensory part, temporal lesions can also occasion *speech disorders* in the absence of sensory defects. Certain mechanisms developed from the sensory come into play in speaking so that disorders of those mechanisms also entail a disorder of speech.

In contrast to the frontal disorders of spontaneous speech, which are mainly associated with reduced performance, there are others in which *quantitative* speech capacity seems initially increased or little changed, but its *quality* is greatly impaired. As mentioned, this is almost exclusively a feature of the temporally (sensory) determined forms.

In some cases, this appears as a kind of *logorrhea,* a flow of words that cannot be stopped nor reduced to writing. (The headlong rush of words described by Oppenheim (1913) no doubt belongs to this category.) In other cases a specific but regularly effective stimulus is required, such as being addressed. In mild cases appearing largely in combination with amnesic aphasia, due to anatomical factors, the logorrhea is occasionally interrupted by hesitation in the search for a word or periphrasis. Another variety that should be mentioned is an abnormal talkativeness, revealing its kinship by occasional linguistic derailments to the paraphasic disorders frequently in association with logorrhea.

In time the accelerated tempo usually decreases, and the whole performance, disregarding these formal defects, sometimes resembles a well-delivered speech in a foreign language, a resemblance heightened by the usually preserved intonational pattern.

The form of this speech flow, so far as the motor act is concerned, does not appear to be disturbed. However, apart from the above talkativeness, it is qualitatively altered in the most varied ways by paraphasic disturbances. Depending on whether the word or its components are affected, we distinguish a *verbal paraphasia* (confusion of words) and a *literal* or *syllabic paraphasia* (distortion of words). In the first form a wrong word, which often comes from the normal vocabulary, appears in place of the correct word. At times, words of similar sound take the place of the correct word. In the other form, there are transpositions, insertions, and omissions of syllables or letters, which in severe cases of word distortion result in conglomerates of letters that cannot be disentangled; this is also termed "jargon aphasia." These disturbances resemble in part the effect of articulatory disorders described in motor aphasia and for that reason are also designated as paraphasic. However, there is a different tempo; in the one, there is rapid, smooth, uninterrupted "derailment," often with no insight into the pathology of the whole; in the other, toiling, groping effort with constant awareness of failure. The verbal and literal forms may occur together and mixed from the beginning. In milder cases, undistorted phrases and letters are interwoven. Here again, the phenomena differ according to the difficulty and familiarity of what is to be said, accounting for the fact that well-practiced series are more or less intact. The sentence melody apparently is always preserved. Sometimes the paraphasia is noted only in naming objects and is absent in the rest of speech. Also of importance in explaining the phenomena is that even in cases of severe spontaneous paraphasia, reading may sometimes be correct, and imitative singing will sometimes ameliorate the paraphasia. Correct copying makes no change in the accompanying literal paraphasia.

The patient's insight into the disorder varies; in milder cases, it is evidenced by attempts at self-correction which occassionally succeed, but it is often lacking until the late stable stage, so that the patient only notices the deficient effect of the jargon. Awareness of the disorder sometimes leads to intentional silence. An important clinical and localizing feature is the occasional sudden onset of paraphasic logorrhea in motor aphasic cases, obviously a complication.

Pathogenetically related to the phenomena under discussion, though apparently representing only a modified repetition of what is heard, *echolalia* should be mentioned here (Pick, 1916; Liepmann, 1900). It consists in its most severe form in an immediate, compulsive and irresistible (Wernicke) imitation of everything spoken, often to the most minute articulatory and musical detail, even of utterances not understood, foreign languages, long chemical formulae, or meaningless sequences of letters (in fresh and severe cases sometimes with complete exclusion of spontaneous speech). Or it may occur as a partial echo, either of the last parts of words or more rarely the beginning of what is heard. In a mitigated from, as the disorder begins to improve, it is restricted at first to a questioning repetition of what is said to the patient; later, it occurs as an adaptation to the patient's own speech; the speech intention, which is maintained against the compulsion to imitate, is immediately followed by the answer to what has been said, though early in the disorder, often with logorrhea and paraphasic distortions. With gradual improvement the tempo as well as the compulsiveness is moderated, although sometimes a tendency to repeat is detectable for a long time, definitely influencing spontaneous speech. In rarer cases, a slow echolalia, similar in every respect to voluntary repetition, will persist for some time. In cases of idiocy, echolalia is occasionally the highest stage of speech development. When the intelligence is intact, persistant echolalia can be overcome, as can other standstills in speech development. We should also mention as pertinent for this account the echoing of nonliguistic utterances of the speech mechanism (musical signals) and the association with other echo phenomena (echographia, echopraxia).

Except for some traces persisting in normals, the acoustic motor reflex is subject to inhibition by voluntary speech and the higher processes, a fact important for the interpretation of echolalia. As a result of a usually focal lesion (in the temporal lobe, usually including and more rarely excluding Wernicke's zone) there is suppression of inhibition, hence disinhibition of the reflex, and echolalia. Milder forms correspond to gradual reactivation and reinforcement of the inhibition or to deactivation of the disinhibitory effect on speech initiative. This appears in speech as a conflict between the compulsion to speak arising from disinhibition and the speech intention. In rare cases, when the residual echolalia exhibits the character of voluntary repetition, the compulsion to repeat still seems at times to be effective. Perhaps this is the result of a learned attunement to such a reaction under certain conditions. In severe cases, when no linguistically intelligible speech is produced but rhythm and intonation are recognizable in the echolalia, there is reversion to the pre-speech stage of the child, in which the speech melody heard is transferred into babbling.

As patients will testify, logorrhea must also be considered a disinhibition, chiefly affecting the tempo of the otherwise undisturbed utterance. However, in such cases it is mainly the quality of speech that appears to be disturbed by the frequent combination with paraphasia.

The explanation of the disorders of disinhibition is based upon the differentiation of their effects into confusion of words and distortion of words, which make it a priori probable that this distinction is due to the onset of the disturbance at different stages in the speech process. The former concerns the stage of word choice (not a very apt expression, since the process is an automatic one), as confirmed by the juxtaposition and interchange of words in milder cases (otitic abscess of the temporal lobe, operation in that region), and by the self-admitted conflict of amnestic and verbal paraphasic phenomena. Clinically, the former, i.e. the absence of the anticipated word in the flow of speech, differs from verbal paraphasia in that word amnesia is characterized by an inhibition of the inappropriate word, founded on the intention toward the correct word (Selz, 1922), which in the verbal paraphasia does not suffice. In milder cases, attempts at correction occur during the flow of speech as a result of awareness of error. (Something of the kind also occurs in functional aphasic disorders accompanying migraine.) In *verbal paraphasia,* the word determined by thoughts and by the sentence pattern is inwardly present or at least there is an intention in this direction, but this normally rigid determination is loosened up. The coherence is not firm enough to maintain the normal suppression of words evoked by association from the sphere of meaning, from parallel lines of thought, or by other sorts of confusion, and it thus leads to the transmission of one of the inapposite words to the speech mechanism. Similiarities of words, parts of words, and word combinations, may also play a part. The effect of the intact part of the speech process (especially the sentence pattern) on the wrong word is sometimes evidenced in the word as a grammatical modification derived from the correct word, but incorrect when used with the paraphasia. In milder cases, the patient, like the amnesiac, immediately recognizes the correct word when offered and uses it appropriately. This interpretation is supported by the fact that the patient is often aware of the compulsiveness of the whole process, as in the embarrassment which follows his blurting out of the wrong word. At times, the whole process is felt by the patient as compulsive and therefore humorous. That thought normally precedes speech probably plays a role, in that the relaxation of the coherence no longer prevents the shifting to a different complex.

That this loosening of coherence does not affect all parts of the inwardly formulated sentence is shown by the fact that except for the most severe cases, the sentence and intonational pattern remain undisturbed, so that the loosening must affect the subsequent stages of the speech process.

The rigidity produced psychologically by determination is probably matched by a physiological tension from above.

Disinhibition is also a causal factor in word distortion, a purely descriptive term for *literal paraphasia*. Here the defect obviously affects the structure of individual words, and since the motor apparatus itself is intact, it must be assumed to involve the successive elicitation of its functions; i.e. in the regulatory action of the transmission mechanism which must be impaired by disinhibition with respect to sound sequences.

According to our knowledge of normal slips of the tongue, the separate forms of the disorder may be explained as anteception, metaception, postception, and paraception (Meringer and Mayer, 1895; Saint-Paul, 1909). To these may be added contamination and perseveration. The not infrequent mixture of verbal and literal paraphasia presumably corresponds to the simultaneous occurrence of disinhibition in both the stages in question.

There is also a second causal factor. In severe cases with combined verbal and literal paraphasia, the word-deafness by which they are usually accompanied is a result of a disturbance in the acoustic portion of the inner word. The function of the transmission mechanism is impaired in relation to the normal guiding role of the acoustic element in speech. This appears most clearly in literal paraphasia and jargon aphasia.

The logorrhea which often occurs in such cases may be due to the acceleration and perhaps also to the temporal shift between thinking and speaking. This is supported by the occurrence of paraphasic-like disorders in connection with flights of ideas and language, as normal rapid speech will promote slips of the tongue. In such cases, the disinhibition or the loosening of coherence which underlies it is at an earlier stage of the process. The starting point for our interpretation, taken from the combination of paraphasic and amnestic phenomena, is supported by the fact that improvement in the paraphasic component leads to a return to the stage of the amnestic, i.e. hesitation due to lack of the correct word, as compared to the previous uninhibited utterance of incorrect words. Let us note particularly that according to this view, the lack of accelerated tempo, especially in the later stages, offers no evidence against the interpretation given here.

Lastly, incorrect distribution of attention may also play a part, since distraction brings about slips of the tongue even in normal individuals, apparently as a result of a diminished inhibition.

The correctness of this view of the literal form resulting from disinhibition in the stage of word formation is confirmed by the observation of speech products in epileptic aura *(uf, uf, nek, jak, ef, jo, dol, ko)*, where disinhibition probably attains its highest degree. The occasional seizure-like occurrence of paraphasia in connection with epileptic attacks, especially those that are determined by temporal cortical lesions, also lends support to this interpretation. These relationships of logorrhea and paraphasia to the psychic processes have their anatomical basis in the fact that in the temporal epileptic "dreamy states" of H. Jackson, flights of ideas commonly occur along with paraphasic and amnestic phenomena.

Differences in self-awareness of the disorder, apart from the realization that the utterance meets with no response from the listener, can be explained by the varying attitude of the patient while putting his thoughts into speech (whether focusing on pronunciation or content).

Early interpretations of paraphasia based on the loss of a regulative function for speech associated with the acoustic speech center in T1, as proposed by Wernicke, are refuted by the fact that this condition occurs in cases of temporal lesion without involvement of that center. It has also been established, contrary to previous opinion, that hearing oneself does not provide such control, since one does not ordinarily listen to his own speech.

Another previous interpretation based on insufficient attention, derived from observations on normal slips of the tongue, appears partially justified, inasmuch as deficient attention or improper distribution of attention entails a relaxation of normal inhibitions; but this does not alter the fact that in paraphasia, attention directed toward the effect often worsens the disorder. However, disordered attention might be effective since, as discussed, it might also loosen up the coherence.

The occurrence of paraphasia with bilateral lesion of Wernicke's zone proves that it is not a function of the right hemisphere in compensation for inactivation of the left.

Liepmann (1914) interprets the various forms of disturbance in paraphasia (anteception and postception, fusions) by means of a defective "acoustic model." This is assumed in analogy with his interpretation of apraxia. Apart from objections to this model, which will not be discussed here, it should be noted that while this explanation accounts for the form of the phenomena (again, the acoustic portion of inner speech is assumed to be involved), it does not reveal the fundamental mechanisms.

Occasionally, correct rote speaking occurs along with paraphasia. This is explained by the fact that motor structures, firmly established by practice, are unimpaired by disinhibition in the higher mechanisms, or at least not impaired in constant fashion, as seen in the derailments which occur now and then. Correct reading or repetition of speech may be explained by the resistance to derailments afforded by concentration on writing or heard speech, i.e. by the establishment of an artificial form of inhibition through the formation of an effective coherence pattern.

The frequent and marked discrepancy between paraphasia and paragraphia is similarly explained. The coherence between speaking and writing, so firm in normals, is also loosened up, so that an opportunity is afforded for additional derailments of this sort; moreover, it is much the same with paralexia, in cases where the coherence established by seeing the printed word is inadequate.

Paraphasic naming of objects in the absence of the same disorder in spontaneous speech corresponds to the greater difficulty of object-naming, which brings out the otherwise latent defect, a relationship found also in paragraphia without paraphasia.

Regarding the etiology, both contamination of ideas and contamination of language may lead to similar paraphasic defects of a verbal and literal nature. This suggests that this factor may be involved in nonparaphasic disorders as well. The possibility must also be considered that disorders of attention may also lead to defective continuation of the ongoing sentence, both as to content and construction.

Emphasis on the significance of this inhibition as presented here helps to align paraphasia with other phenomena attributed to this factor, such as echolalia and logorrhea.

This relationship may be understood as follows: echolalia of sudden onset is the most severe form, whereby volition is either entirely eliminated or not effective after the disorder improves; the second is logorrhea in its various modifications, whereby words flow out uninhibitedly, either undistorted or with occasional verbal displacements; the third form is verbal paraphasia; and the fourth, literal paraphasia with word distortion. In other words, disinhibition first occurs without essential disturbance of the inner structure, which only takes place later. The differentiation of the various forms clearly suggests that the disinhibited areas must also differ. The fact that all occur predominantly with lesion of the temporal lobe (ordinarily on the left side) is explained by the fact that mechanisms relating to the inhibiting functions are combined with the speech mechanisms at that precise location, so that lesion of these areas will produce a selective and comprehensive effect. As mentioned, similar effects can also be produced by lesion in a region to which that area is (functionally) subordinate.

Since the analogous phenomena thus produced are usually of a mild degree, it is conceivable that the inhibition arises in areas so large as to overcome the disinhibition provoked by focal lesion. Consistent with this interpretation is the fact that in the presumably functional disease of tic, as in similar syndromes regarded as having an anatomical basis (e.g. eclampsia), there are abundant disinhibitions (ed. release phenomena) in the form of echopraxia, echomimia, and echographia. Little can be added regarding other anatomical regions, except to note that the frontal lobe is claimed to be an inhibiting organ, a view that appears incorrect at least for the speech field, since similar forms of disinhibition have not been observed in isolation with frontal lesions. Should such phenomena occur, which must be very rare indeed, they may be interpreted as due to concurrent anatomical or functional involvement of the temporal portion of the speech field.

It should also be remarked that previous views of excitation as a causal factor in these disinhibitory phenomena have now been generally abandoned (Oppenheim, 1913), for the main reason that apart from the typicality of the phenomena, identical disturbances are absent in lesions of Broca's area.

Nor can we accept the assumption that echolalia differs from logorrhea in its more greatly reduced intention (Goldstein). This cannot account for the mitigated forms of echolalia, as explained through disinhibition, as in the immediate reappearance of intention when the disinhibition subsides. The extension of echo phenomena to other modalities of the speech mechanism, such as musical and other symbols, even in late stages also speaks against the assumption that intention plays a part.

That these forms of disinhibition are not a regular consequence of focal lesion in the designated areas has not yet been explained. However, it shows that we are concerned here with functional effects of the lesions, while other more or less permanent disorders reflect the local damage caused by the lesions. This is supported by the diminution of the disinhibitions, echolalia first, the others in order, logorrhea being the most persistent. This corresponds to the interpretation of these phenomena as the expression of still other causal factors. Accordingly, the following may be said in regard to foci in the temporal lobe: it is a common clinical observation in progressive lesions affecting this region, e.g. in tumors which arise in the mesocranial fossa and grow upward toward the temporal lobes, that the sequence of phenomena is word amnesia, verbal paraphasia with occasional logorrhea, literal paraphasia, and finally word-deafness. This sequence of disinhibitory phenomena can only be explained by the varying functional effect of the lesion, while for other symptoms, as yet undefined anatomical differences may play a decisive role.

The reason why some cases have awareness of the disorder and others do not is unknown. In addition to the patient's observation of the lack of response to his utterance, other psychic factors play a part, including self-deception based upon the retained sentence and intonational pattern.

Regarding the genetic relationship of paraphasia and sensory paragrammatism asserted by some authors, see the discussion of paragrammatism below.

A similar phenomenon formerly classed as echolalia because it is also due to disinhibition should be noted here in passing, namely *palilalia*. Although occasionally spontaneous, it more often consists of a reactive autorepetition of the same word or short sentence, in an echolalic-like manner, often up to eight to ten times in succession; it is somewhat explosive and often accelerates with an increasingly rising tone. It has recently been shown (Pick, 1921) to possibly be a subordinate phenomenon of a disinhibition determined by the extrapyramidal system.

Chapter 11

PERSEVERATION

A<small>T THIS POINT</small>, because of a similar pathogenesis, another distinct condition should be mentioned. Though not totally absent in other functional forms (even in the field of apraxia), it plays a major role in connection with the above aphasic phenomena and appears mainly with disorders resulting from lesion of the temporal lobe (usually on the left side). This has to do with "perseveration," in which a functional form which is ordinarily supplanted by the next in succession persists unaltered and leads repeatedly to the same product, or *perseverate*. This should not be confused with the residual formulae of the motor aphasic, which persist for a long time and without change. Presumably, we are dealing here with an intensification of a phenomenon found in normals, viz. a word already used either reappears or has a further effect in the sentence. This is also seen in the normal phenomenon of slips of the tongue. Pathological perseveration appears in just this form as a part of the disorders under discussion: in word amnesia as the urgent and often multiple repetition of the same word distortion or word confusion, as the continued effect of a previous sentence construction or word inflection, occasionally simulating agrammatism; in contrast, the correct grammatical construction of the perseverated word or the perseverated false intonation of a correct word shows that the disorder affects only a part of an otherwise intact process. It is often hard to furnish proof of this relationship, since only the final perseverate is available for appraisal. We must delve into the psychic to explain why the patient answers "thirty-one" when asked how many children he has, when the previous question was about his marriage thirty-one years past, the date of which was not discussed. There are other ways that a word called to mind may appear as a perseverate. A patient whose state of health has been previously discussed will produce the same word without change when asked the names of objects. Similar phenomena are found in reading and writing; in the latter, the more difficult task, even when perseveration has otherwise disappeared. In writing, there is also perseveration derived from speech (after "Spiel" appears "sbischbiel"). One patient writes "getorito potogeto geriti."

This obviously functional disorder may extend over many days with long free intervals, as after paralytic and epileptic attacks, especially those involving the temporal lobes. Ordinarily the left side is concerned, although the phenomenon may be observed in connection with right-sided lesions, even in the absence of left-handedness. The nature of the disorder is not well known. There is justification, on the basis of the norm, and for at least some cases, for the assumption (von Solder) that the intense after effect is due to an action reinforced by attention and interest. However, in the pathological case, the inadequacy of certain actions in consequence of fatigue or lowered level of awareness results in prominence of the perseveration. This is supported by the paradigmatic nature of the phenomenon, even normals in states of reduced capacity, and particularly under conditions of extreme fatigue.

The frequent concomitance of perseveration with paraphasia due to temporal lesion and resulting from disinhibition suggests that similar immediate causative factors may be concerned in the origin of perseveration. This is probably true. It is a common observation (Stransky, 1905) that acceleration of speech easily and regularly leads to perseveration. Moreover, the weakness of coherence and determination which are assumed to explain paraphasia correspond to the reduction in other capacities unrelated to the perseverate which have been postulated in order to explain perseveration. The parallel phenomenon of fatigue derived from normals has also been occasionally observed to result in speech disinhibition with paraphasia. It is surely no accident that in both instances it is in the search for words that relaxation of coherence leads to such evident disinhibitions; surely, the relevant difficulty of the performance must play a part.

In addition, there is the factor of localization, which also speaks in favor of the close association between the two, evidenced by the fact that in rare organic cases acute paraphasia and perseveration occur together as in the aforementioned "attacks."

Since it can hardly be conjectured that the disorder underlying perseveration is restricted to the temporal lobes, it must be assumed that temporal disinhibitions bring about its appearance. We cannot ignore the fact that impressive processes also localized in the temporal lobes reveal nothing corresponding to perseveration, though this may be merely apparent, since the patient is unable to testify in this regard. In certain forms of word deafness, when patients say that everything they hear seems monotonous and uniform, e.g. "toterot" or "drub-arub-drub," an impressive perseveration may be involved.

Chapter 12

REPETITION AND ROTE SPEECH

V<small>OLUNTARY REPETITION</small> takes place either directly, *without regard to comprehension,* by use of the remnants of the primitive speech reflex which leads to a state of readiness of the corresponding motor centers which facilitiates the repetition, or indirectly, *by way of the more or less incipient understanding of what has been said.* Clinically, it usually corresponds closely with the quality of spontaneous speech. In aphemia, repetition is often lacking, so that even formulae (ed. stereotypies, cliches) cannot be repeated. Perfectly correct repetition may be seen in rare instances, though mild ideations are more usual, as in paraphasia, as previously mentioned. When spontaneous speech is fluent repetition is generally better, since it is an easier performance, though occasionally with variations of individual letters and incorrect intonation. In cases with agrammatism, repetition is usually also agrammatical. The converse, repetition that is worse than spontaneous speech, is an exception. Repetition of longer words and sentences depends on comprehension and attention; the former augments while the latter detracts if attention span is diminished. Repetition can also be found in the absence of speech comprehension, for it is not dependent on the latter. Of course, the loss of sound perception will severely disturb repetition. If grammatical comprehension is impaired, even when there is no agrammatism of spontaneous speech, repetition may be agrammatical and defective. When the pronunciation of perceived speech is correct, this may occur as a result of its inadequate reconstruction.

Often long words are repeated better than sentences of the same length and better than isolated letters or syllables. The effect of the varying degree of success in comprehension usually appears in the better repetition of meaningful words than meaningless ones. The same is true of attempts to reproduce, with the aid of incidental and meaningful associations, sentences that cannot be independently reproduced in a meaningful manner. Lip reading also helps; it is very quickly learned by many patients and improves performance on repetition tests.

That the quality of repetition generally keeps pace with that of speech is understandable because those factors which impair spontaneous speech also influence repetition. However, in immediate repetition, their effect is ameliorated by the motor attunement to perceived speech, as mentioned above. The rare phenomenon of inferior repetition is probably determined by the loss of this attunement and also by other poorly understood functional factors which differ in the individual case (improper adjustment of attention toward the motor act itself, for example). As an aggravating circumstance we may consider the fact that repetition is an act of will, a task, which directly occasions attention to its result, and in cases where the result is poor, attention has a particularly deleterious effect. That what is understood is as a rule repeated better than what is not understood results from the advantage offered to excitation of the speech apparatus by sentence meaning and inner-speech associated with the individual words.

Concerning the anatomical basis for retained repetition in the presence of disordered speech comprehension, partial lesion of Wernicke's area or a lesion in the vicinity, nothing can be said with certainty. It should be noted, however, that repetition without comprehension is an achievement entirely alien to normal life and for that reason difficult. The effort made to extract meaning from meaningless words will further impair the performance. Since the meaning is normally attributed to what is spoken, and the examinee does not always have a conscious mental set in this regard, this will further add to the difficulty of meaningless repetition.

It is premature to correlate these diverse symptoms with specific anatomical findings, not only because of our deficient anatomical knowledge (intracortical paths) but also because of the complexity of the situation (participation of the right hemisphere?). In general it is chiefly the arcuate fasciculus that is anatomically involved in repetition, along with other association fibers between the temporal and frontal regions.

Among the speech forms favored by an intensive development of motor structures over long series (an aspect that plays a part in ordinary speaking as well) is the so-called *rote speech,* the recitation of automatized sequences of words and sentences, of prayers, the multiplication table, the names of the days of the week and months of the year, school verses, and so on. This includes the factor of age (what is learned in youth being retained better than what is acquired later) and places this speech form among those most strongly resistant to focal lesions.

The tempo of the phenomenon varies, depending on other defects, but not always in comparable degree. (Even in severe aphemia rote speech may be rapid.) The supreme importance of functional connections firmly established through practice is proved by the inability to resume the series once interrupted without starting again from the beginning and also the inability to immediately correct an error in the series. Here again we are confronted with the opposition between volition and automatism discussed in detail above, as when a bit of dialect may suddenly appear in the midst of rote speaking. The effect of practice will vary, sometimes there is rapid reestablishment, sometimes repeated failure.

Embolophasia is a phenomenon in this class in which certain expletives are inserted into speech, usually without the patient's awareness. As in normals, a formula is accidentally established and then automatized, which like rote speech often has the effect in cases of lowered speech capacity of mobilizing an otherwise impossible sentence by way of the expletive. Similarly, the entire series is more frequently mobilized if the examiner runs through it first or simply indicates the start. In recovery it is occasionally observed that practice in one series initiates others unpracticed.

Rote speaking represents still a more highly automatized form of an already strongly automatized function. Accordingly, all that has been said regarding the effects of practice will serve to explain the greater resistance of rote speech compared to spontaneous speech. In addition, there is the facilitated stimulation of the automatic and extensive motor structures, with concomitant reduction of the effect of volition required for their excitation. The rigid coherence of the motor structures established by practice explains the inability to begin in the middle of them and the mobilization of a series or a part of a series by the insertion of an activating cue word, by repetition or by singing. In the last instance, in addition to the structural coherence, there is the relationship, fixed through practice, between the structures of music and lyric, of which the former is especially well established.

Obviously this also applies with modification to retraining after the loss of a function. These factors, especially the frequent contrast between total aphemia and good rote speaking, speak in favor of this interpretation and especially against the assumption of anarthria. Moreover, the fact that practice of one series carries over to others speaks against the assumed loss of memory images. Nor can this result entirely from the rhythm of a series, since each series has its own rhythm; it is more likely due to the improved mobility and plasticity of the corresponding groups of neurons, just as a violinist if forced to play the piano will at first play better than one who has never played. It is obvious that psychic factors, such as pleasure in the results, also play a part.

Chapter 13

WORD AMNESIA (AMNESTIC APHASIA) AND OPTIC APHASIA

THE SPEECH DISORDER which appears in the absence or lack of recall for the proper word in the process of object naming or in the course of a sentence has a special importance. It is now established that this disorder, *word amnesia,* which for a long time was denied as a distinct clinical form, can persist over a long time as the only symptom, therefore justifying its position as *a separate form of aphasia, amnestic aphasia.* In this disorder, the word corresponding to the idea does not emerge, and the patient, after expressing his inability in some way, tries for a substitute in paraphrase or by indicating the purpose of the object, but when even a fragment of the word is suggested to the patient, he immediately recognizes it and can reproduce it correctly. The phenomenon occurs as a symptom variably affecting the naming of objects when spontaneous speech does not yet show any sign of word amnesia. In severe cases, it is occasionally followed by inability to indicate the purpose of the object. Seeing the object usually facilitates naming, but occasionally touch is also necessary. The disorder first affects substantives, primarily proper names and abstract words, more rarely verbs and adjectives, almost never prepositions and articles (see under agrammatism). All other parts of the speech process, and particularly the stages of formulation, are completely undisturbed with the exception of tempo, which though intact and lively, will be interrupted by the inability to find a particular word. In polyglots as a rule, the last acquired language first shows word amnesia.

The word amnesia that occurs mainly in older persons is to some extent analogous to this disorder, as well as states of fatigue and exhaustion. Besides this pure amnestic aphasia, the same phenomenon is found side by side with other aphasic disorders, especially the sensory aphasias, a relationship which appears clinically in the fact that a pure or almost amnestic aphasia commonly persists—at times indefinitely—as a residual of a marked sensory aphasia. Conversely, in progressive cases, amnestic aphasia may represent the first stage of a disorder which later more clearly exhibits symptoms of a sensory form of aphasia. In the same way, it may be the manifestiation of an early stage of a more widespread disease of the cortex (general paralysis, senile dementia). The early involvement of the left temporal lobe in atrophic processes, which has not yet been fully explained, probably plays the major role here. Symptoms which are similar in nature to those of sensorily determined amnestic aphasia are also found, though more rarely, as remnants of a motor aphasia, but in these cases some hint of the underlying motor speech disturbance is evident.

This interpretation should be prefaced by the remark that in the normal course of speech there is no real search or selection of the appropriate words. Instead, this process takes place automatically, though less than other components of the speech process which occur mainly via the feeling for the language *(Sprachgefühl)*. Because of these factors "word-finding" is one of the more difficult speech functions and is therefore more vulnerable, even in diffuse and functional conditions.

This is even more true of tests of object-naming during an examination, for it is an artificial situation and not to be compared with the use of single words that really does occur (the one-word *sentence*). The impromptu quality of this performance without any aid (dictionary) helps to explain its difficulty. It calls for a special achievement of signification. In the choice of words in the sentence, it is not a simple association of the name with the object that is involved, but a process of fitting the selected word to the meaning of the entire sentence (apart, of course, from the use of familiar formulae and trite expressions). This performance is still more complex with regard to other categories of words.

Object naming in order to convey meaning concerns a learned or affectively conditioned function, which is therefore performed more readily. During speech, various aids are provided by the sentence context, especially since logical memory is undisturbed. The restriction of the disturbance to certain categories of words is based on their functional grouping, more or less according to the difficulty and familiarity of the underlying psychological and/or physiological processes. There is no simple answer to this question, since variations may arise from altered functional conditions (different stages of the speech process). For this reason, the problem cannot be solved only by the consideration of various word categories, as often done in the derivation of Ribot's rule.

The earlier involvement of object naming over object definition or description is due to a difference in development. The designation of objects is a latter acquisition and therefore is less resistant than the indication of their use. The name has been added to the properties of the thing and is therefore not so inherent as its properties. A related phenomenon is the greater ability to indicate the object when given the name than to supply the name when presented the object. Early in development the object and its use are synonymous. (The priority of the action concept over the object concept remains. A thing is primarily an occasion for activity; compare also onomatopoetica, which, since it is derived from the function, represents the object more directly than the conventional name.)

In explanation of this fact, Selz (1922) assumes that when memory dispositions of words are weakened, their excitation by the object or the concept fails. This is clearly in harmony with the older interpretation of amnestic aphasia based on a slight attenuation of the acoustic memory images. It also corresponds to the localization, but is of course valid only for the names of objects, since other factors come into consideration for other categories of words.

The greater difficulty of abstract nouns than concrete ones in due to the fact that the former are understood through relational experiences, while the latter are known from perception. The relational experiences are less available than the known elements of perception and must be at least partially reproduced. Proper names are also produced more readily since they do not have etymological relationships to other familiar words.

This dynamic interpretation derived from phenomena corresponds to an analysis of the underlying processes. Patients will indicate the loss of the acoustic inner speech component or call attention to the fact that such loss prevents excitation of motor speech processes. In severe cases, the occurrence of paraphasic symptoms (for this combination see under paraphasia) argues for the intactness of inner speech in word amnesia and is consistent with the notion of impaired motor-speech stimulation.

We may consider the failure of the intended word to emerge as an expression of its unreadiness for reproduction as prompted by the idea or the object. Thus, the reactiveness of this component is readily aroused when the word is heard, this stimulus being most adequate since both are ontogenetically old and share a precise mutual attunement. Stimulation of the acoustic component by other speech processes, such as reading, is facilitated by the coherence of the concerned inner speech factors. There are varying degrees of this disorder; a mild form occurs when a structure corresponding to the missing word is produced before the word itself emerges. This suggests a coherence of those processes, the relaxation of which was previously held to be the cause of paraphasic derailments.

Through psychological analysis it can be shown that typical pure amnestic aphasia is related to the sequence of the processes in sentence formation. Clinical observation localizes the disorder mainly to the sensory portion of the speech field (in initial cases almost exclusively) as demonstrated in many cases and confirmed by autopsy findings. This concerns lesions in the second and third temporal convolutions, ordinarily on the left side; in those rare instances of right-sided lesions one must assume a functional influence in the homologous areas of the left side. Diffuse affectations of the cerebral cortex may show a relatively greater involvement of these areas. This suggests that the temporal lobe plays the prominent role here also by an involvement of a "concept field" (Goldstein), but probably related to other associated phenomena. It is not certain in cases of relatively pure amnestic aphasia due to motor aphasia to what extent a functional influence on the temporal regions of the speech field must be assumed. In these cases, a disturbance of conductance from the inner-speech transmission mechanism to the motor-speech center may be involved. At times, depending on the linguistic type of the patient, particularly with regard to foreign languages, a component different from that discussed is involved in the impairment of word-finding, namely the acoustic component of inner speech. This would explain the indirect effect of distant lesions.

It follows that the localization of amnestic aphasia does not concern a "center for names" but rather the determination of a region from which impairment most easily arises in those processes which parallel the observed psychological processes. Involvement of the lower parietal lobe, as postulated by Goldstein, does not have adequate clinical and patho-anatomical foundation.

For the sake of completeness, two other disorders should be mentioned here. First, the so-called *optic* or *visual aphasia* by which term Freund implied a patient who, unable to name an object seen, immediately produces the name on touching or otherwise perceiving the object, while in other cases the correct word does not emerge even in this way (hearing or touching the object). It has been thought that a *tactile aphasia* might be assumed in cases where palpation does not elicit the name which is produced by other means.

We are concerned here (ignoring a possible impairment of perception, which occasionally gives rise to errors) with differences in reactiveness of the acoustic portion of inner speech regarding the various stimuli coming from the object.

However it may be with such observations, in any case rare, there can be no doubt that these are not varieties of disease but are functionally determined phenomena. They are not regularly associated with a specific locus, but along with other similar phenomena, so far as visual aphasia is concerned, relate to the boundary region between temporal and occipital lobes.

It is necessary to emphasize again what has been said about the artificiality of testing methods.

Secondly, the disturbance termed *"color-name amnesia"* should be mentioned, which is observed in amnestic aphasics. It consists not only of inability to name colors in spite of intact color vision but also of disorders in sorting wool samples, which on casual inspection may suggest impaired color vision. Patients also have difficulty indicating the colors of objects perceived or demonstrating them on color samples. It has now been established, especially by the evidence of correct periphrasis (Head), that the phenomenon has no relation to color concepts (Goldstein, Head). Similar observations in children (Peters, 1915), indicate that the *name* of the color plays an intermediate role in sorting and usually also in searching for the color of the perceived object. The need for speech in these functions accounts for the disorder as a consequence of amnesia for color names, which are poorly understood even when heard and read. Head has demonstrated that lesions result in a similar impairment in other functions or their expression in language as a result of a semantic disturbance requiring the aid of speech.

Also we should mention parenthetically that patients who can use letters correctly may not know how to pronounce their names, but immediately recognize the letters when their names are pronounced. This does not resolve even with general improvement. Again we see a contrast between good automatic performance, in consequence of intact structures, and poor performance with respect to their parts.

Chapter 14

AGRAMMATISM

Among the phenomena of motor aphasia, some were discussed which appear in the loss of or disturbance in the use of those linguistic devices which in a general way serve to grammaticize speech. We shall now discuss this form together with some others.

The descriptive terms which have been applied to these various forms are partly derived from anatomical and partly from functional considerations. They have only gradually become known, having been initially grouped together under the designation agrammatism. To eliminate the obscurities which arise from this fact we must add a few remarks on the nomenclature.

The term was first used in a general way for agrammatism of presumably frontal origin. When it was found to occur with a lesion of the temporal (sensory) portion of the speech field, a *sensory agrammatism* was distinguished from what had been termed *motor agrammatism* because of its association with motor aphasia. Following this, it was observed that in the *impressive* part of speech, in speech comprehension, defects in the comprehension of grammatical form occur which deserve to be included in agrammatism and are thus designated sensory.

Moreover, the recognition that temporally determined expressive agrammatism is characterized by erroneous grammatical constructions (paragrammatisms) in contrast to the frontal type with its *telegraphic style* led Kleist to distinguish the temporal form as *paragrammatism*.

Since we have already discussed the symptomatology of motor agrammatism let us now, with regard to pathogenesis, approach the pertinent defects of the expressive side with a comparable description of paragrammatism.

This temporally determined form is characterized, in pure cases, by disturbances in the use of auxiliary words, incorrect word inflections, and erroneous prefixes and suffixes. In other words, it concerns all those linguistic devices which serve to express *relationships* between objects, which differ widely and numerically from one language to another. According to the localization, other temporal symptoms are found in the early stages which may later disappear. In contrast to motor agrammatism, the tempo of speech is not retarded, tending rather to logorrhea with intact sentence pattern and intonation. Occasionally, some motor (ed. telegrammatic) phenomena are found, such as the dropping of inflections, with juxtaposition of the words that compose the skeleton of the sentence.

In rare cases which, with respect to other symptoms, show complete recovery, and more rarely as an introductory stage in progressive cases, an isolated grammatical disorder may represent the only symptom; e.g. confusion of genders, finally followed by exclusive use of the feminine form.

The patient commonly notices his errors, without always being able to describe or correct them. Occasionally the correct grammatical structure emerges via the feeling for the language evoked by partially saying it aloud to him. The influence of emotions may also have a salutory effect in this case as in others. The frequent coincidence of temporal (expressive) agrammatism with paraphasia, due to the common localization, may result in unintelligible speech, with defects which may be hard to classify. The linguistic formulation plays a guiding role, even in the preparation for writing, and accounts for the occurrence of agrammatism in writing. Also of importance in evaluation is the presence of linguistically justifiable agrammatisms, this being more common in colloquial language than generally supposed, even in highly developed languages (e.g. English).

Any account of the two forms of expressive agrammatism must begin with the clinical fact of a loss or defective command of the grammatical devices of the language (syntax and grammar in the restricted sense). With regard to precise definitions, we must determine how far these phenomena are due to disorders in the speech field and how far they represent secondary phenomena due to disorders in other regions, though surely little can be said about the latter at this time.

Initially, processes of mental and inner-speech formulation preliminary to the speech fields do not appear involved by the particular localization. However, we may infer on the basis of observation that disorders which affect the course of these processes can impair syntax and grammar. Gross disorders of thought in confusion or twilight states, such as mild flights of ideas or thought contamination in manic states, can have such an effect. A manic patient said, "Ich war tödlich Bronchialkatarrh gewesen" (I had been deathly bronchial catarrh). A Czech housemaid unfamiliar with German writes (what has been said of spoken agrammatism also applies to writing) in a hysterical twilight state, *"Kucharko!* Ich bin (inserted later) *klinika* Pick *pripata, chei vam* (unintelligible word marked out) wunschen *a* isst *zavreli."**

These factors can obviously also affect word order in different ways. Whether this is also true of organic lesions sparing the speech field is the subject of a study undertaken by Head. It is, for example, probable that disorders of the linguistic representation of spatial relationships may be due to spatial disorders, as in defects of orientation, which because of defective formulation of thought entail a defective use of the corresponding auxiliary words. Also we must consider the fact that the patient stresses significant words reflecting his emotional state and not the situation as seen by the listener, and this may make speech unintelligible to the listener.

These factors fall outside the strict field of aphasia, and it is not always possible to determine whether their influence also concerns or involves the speech field processes under consideration. However, there may also be factors within aphasia proper which are also active in the process of thought and speech formulation. Among those already mentioned as more frequent are the narrowness of the perspective of awareness, in part the unpurposeful distribution of attention (regarded by Kussmaul as the sole cause of agrammatism) and incongruences between formulation in thought and formulation in language (with resultant thought and speech contaminations). Nor is it unlikely that the above speech production could be secondarily

---

**Editor's note:* The words written here in italics are Czech, the rest German, except for the bracketed portions which represent the author's interpolated notes. Translation: *"Cook!* I have been *admitted* (without conjugation) Pick *clinic* (nominative), I *want to* wish *you and* is *they have locked me in."*

impaired by other disorders of the speech field. Thus, defective verbal memory may impair the syntactical structure, since another word put in the place of the missing one may have a damaging effect on the sentence construction.

Regarding telegraphic style of primary origin, discussed in relation to motor agrammatism, in which the word order is not appreciably disturbed, alterations of word order have occasionally been reported as due to a discrepancy between the normal order (most important element first) and the grammatically required order (final position of the verb as in the languages of children). However, a thorough investigation of this question, based upon linguistics, the language of children, deaf-mutes and sign language, is not yet available. As in normals, the condition is due to the fact that the intention is chiefly directed towards that meaning which is expressed primarily by nouns and verbs, so that the words which form the skeleton of the sentence are stressed while the accompanying auxiliary words which are thought or felt remain unuttered. We see this in the situation where the patient strongly believes he has spoken the omitted words. In regard to word order, we must also consider the opposing influences of emotion and the preserved feeling for the language. Certain disturbances of this kind (e.g. verb at the end of the sentence) represent the reversion to a childish mode of speech. In discussing defective processes of grammatization restricted to the word, we must consider prepositions, word inflection (prefixes and suffixes), articles, and pronouns which serve this purpose. We must also consider the aforementioned effect of practice on these processes, even in the preschool period, which creates a feeling for the language (Sprachgefühl). Consequently, we speak of the analogy of acquired typical linguistic patterns. This feeling for the language surpasses the influence of later grammatical schooling, even in educated persons. (Consideration of this difference is essential in the pertinent examinations.) Laboratory grammaticization of given words and grammaticization in ordinary discourse are by no means the same (grammer and Sprachgefühl!), as observed clinically. In this regard, it should be mentioned that the agrammatical speaker commonly has superior writing. Both the time factor of prolonged formulation and the mental attitude play a part, since for most individuals writing is a considered act. This difference also appears in talking with the doctor and with the family and colleagues. It is readily apparent here that better education is of significance.

In certain cases it must be assumed that auxiliary words, especially prepositions, corresponding to a certain external speech formulation are also lacking in inner speech. More frequently it is not their absence but their inadequate evocation that is responsible for this disorder.

A similar situation applies to word inflection, which is omitted in accordance with the law of economy. This corresponds to normals; the existence of essentially formless languages of high standing (e.g. English) indicates that the corresponding form components in other languages provide an extra that is superfluous to comprehension (cf. also the ordinary telegram!). Conversely, inflection is lacking because it does not adequately or properly respond to the stimulus, leading in the latter case to corresponding errors. In polyglots the disorder will appear in only one langauge or mainly in the latest acquired language.

Testing with single improperly conjugated or declined words, apart from the meaning of the single word as sentence, is chiefly an examination of knowledge gained in school and usually of very brief retention. This appears largely when, in the face of poor test performance, the patient's actual discourse indicates adequate feeling for the language; also, the "formulation of sequences" (Reihenbildung) can be preserved with incorrect word inflection.

A distinction should be made between the above telegraphic style and so-called Negersprache characterized by a simple succession of *uninflected* nouns and verbs. While this form shares with telegraphic style the absence of auxiliary words which characterize relationships, it represents in the dropping of inflectional devices (in certain languages the prefixes and suffixes as well) a still further regression to an infantile stage of speech. It also shares with telegrammatism the fact that relationships are conceived along with the nouns and verbs, or in advance of the utterance, but it shows further regression than telegrammatism.

Regarding the *genesis* of the two forms of expressive agrammatism, a distinction must be made, with reference to *frontal (motor) agrammatism* (the *telegraphic style*) between its immediate onset after a lesion and its slow development with a gradual increase in vocabulary from an initial stage of one-word sentence. In the latter instance, because of the linguistic poverty, a gradual adjustment takes place such that only the skeleton of the sentence is produced. The former instance concerns the factors discussed above: emergence of the skeleton of the sentence alone, during the mental formulation in thought or inner speech; absence of or defect in the auxiliary words which are normally produced in automatic fashion. It is probable that the patient with motor agrammatism at times retains the sentence skeleton since he may not comprehend the prepositions nor be able to write them. We may assume that adjustment to a telegraphic style, which makes the prepositions appear superfluous, will gradually influence formulation in thought. The lack of inflection in juxtaposed words may be explained by speech economy, due to the fact that speech is difficult to produce at all and inflection requires even more energy. The patient attempts to produce the best possible results (that which best makes him understood) with the least expenditure of effort, utilizing the optimal but still automatic application of his linguistic resources. Of the ideas inchoate and ready for transmission to the executive apparatus, only the essential components are selected. (This represents a pathological intensification of what is termed "brachylogy" in linguistic psychology, speech in which the obvious is omitted.) Another likely factor is the attention fixed on the effortful production of speech. If the prepositions are either not automatic or only incompletely so, attention will not suffice for their voluntary production.

This whole line of thought is consistent with the fact that this aphasic disorder concerns an intensification of the normal tendency to agrammatism.

The sentence rhythm will often be intact in cases of advanced recovery, so far as it is subordinate to the retained sentence skeleton. Disturbed rhythm is probably secondary to defective language though a primary impairment may be present due to simultaneous involvement of the corresponding (musical) functional region.

In addition to our previous comments, it should be emphasized that the situation will influence word order, not only the speaker's appraisal of the situation, but what he takes to be the listener's appraisal as well. As a result of his linguistic poverty, the agrammatical patient utilizes the situation far beyond the norm. The relation between spoken and written agrammatism will vary, depending on the mental attitude, whther the patient tends more to the one or the other. Agrammatism may be entirely lacking in writing in spite of the greater difficulty of this performance.

Difficulties will also arise from the conflict between the persistent but ineffectual feeling for sentence form and the forceful influence of emotional factors. This opposition of imitation and spontaneity corresponds to the same phenomena in the speech development of the child.

Isolated words produced in the initial period can be termed agrammatical only, as in the normal case, insofar as they take the place of a sentence. This is evidenced chiefly by observations in which patients speaking in such a manner can modify the few words at their disposal, not only in accent but also in articulation (lala, dada) in the sense of different thoughts.

Parenthetically, we see in the patient's inability to linguistically express the relations of things that disorders directly involving morphology refer back to semiological defects (semantics).

In reeducation, the feeling for the language which results from years of practice plays a part insofar as its remnants can be built upon. Even if one begins grammatical instruction this will not build up a rote sequence, but is effective only as an extension or reconstruction of the feeling of the language.

Awareness of one's defect is commonly lacking in motor agrammatism. As in the normal individual, the patient devotes his attention to the meaning of the uterance. Accordingly, awareness will vary depending on whether he is attending more on speaking (which may lead to further impairment) or trusts to his presumably intact feeling for the language to carry him to success. In many cases the feeling for the language is commonly apparent in the course of the function, and the patient will notice his error. Sometimes he is still unable to specify it, while at other times he hesistates without coming to a conclusion. To some extent this is related to the fact that the patient speaks better with the doctor than in ordinary communication; in the latter case he depends on the established automatism, while in the former the urge toward better speech has a positive effect.

Infantile or *native agrammatism* is an arrest of speech development due to defective brain development or a cerebral disease at a pre-grammatical stage. It is characterized by both frontal and temporal phenomena. In cases of permanent arrest, which may occur independently without other mental defects, proper feeling for the language does not develop, a deficiency which is compensated by later schooling only inadequately if at all. In mentally retarded states the disorder may be due to defective thought formulation, the child not having entered into the "relationship stage," so that relations of things do not properly enter his awareness.

In *paragrammatism,* the *temporal* form of expressive agrammatism, it must be remembered that grammar is by no means a unified process, but contains many factors which may be affected separately or in combination. In this form, the disorder lies one stage deeper than telegrammatism. It is also of a different nature; in the latter, functions corresponding to the inner speech form, which ordinarily are accomplished through the sentence framework, are not carried out (the reasons for this are given above). In the paragrammatical patient, this process, automatized even to the feeling for the language (which is all that is still effective) is accomplished but in a defective manner, since the individual processes occur either improperly or not at all. With regard to the opposition between volition and automatism and the disturbing influence of attention directed toward a function, voluntary intervention in these processes will not be helpful in most cases. Even in normals, as we have shown, grammaticization that relies simply on feeling for the language often succceds better than that directed by the will.

The various paragrammatic errors also concern functionally differentiated degrees of defects in certain forms of activity. This is definitely proven by such observations as isolated confusion of pronouns and more so by the use of *du* retained after an illness in a patient who had evidently used it dialectally in his youth.* Such facts—confusion of *haben* and *sein*†—and forms of the article††—

***Editor's Note:* By this is meant the use of the German familiar pronoun *du* in addressing persons with whom the patient was not on such familiar terms.

†These German equivalents of "have" and "be" are used to form the perfect tenses of different verbs.

††The German article varies for gender, number, and case, not unambiguously,

also show that this is not a disorder of motor function, but a defective application of motor effects. In the normal, these have become automatic through analogies from the feeling of the language and are not carried out on the basis of knowledge of the corresponding grammatical rules. Of course, certain mental processes to which these motor processes are subordinated do come into play.

There is a discrepancy between poor agrammatical speech and better appraisal of ungrammatical sentences presented to the patient. This is explained by the contrast between defective or absent feeling for the language by the fact that the patient recognizes what he sees as incorrect, but is incapable of putting it into correct grammatical form.

This example of a dynamic interpretation clearly demonstrates the advantage over an extremely anatomical view based on assumed "elements" or functions. The assumption of a fixed localization of single words and even parts of words in the neural elements, in explanation of phenomena of the type here discussed, requires us to also assume partial destruction of specific types of discrete ganglionic cells by the lesion.

It is unlikely that temporal expressive agrammatism is an expression of inadequate functioning of the right hemisphere since it occurs with a small lesion. One should be cautious even in the presence of bilateral lesions. Agrammatism due to previous lesion of the left side may reappear or be intensified by symmetrical lesion of the right side. Certainly, the extent to which impairment in interhemispheric relationships is involved must remain in doubt.

The close bonds between the functions affected in amnestic aphasia, paraphasia, and sensory agrammatism are apparent in the freqent concurrence of the three forms and their common localization. Detailed clinical and anatomical research is needed to clarify the relationships and differences between these forms.

Although sensory agrammatism and paraphasia appear to have a common pathogenesis, as suggested by their coincidence and by localizational factors, this does not appear certain, since even in severe

---

but so much more than the noun does that German speakers often think and speak as if its principle function were to distinguish those grammatical categories; in fact, one of the common German names for the article is *das Geschlelechtswort* (the gender word).

paraphasia, components of the sentence form are undisturbed. Moreover, no transitional forms exist between seemingly ungrammatical segments of jargon aphasia and segments with defective forms corresponding to true temporal agrammatism. Therefore, it seems probable that just as paragrammatism is produced by other disorders (thought contamination and sentence contamination), this applies to jargon also as a result of disinhibitions, perhaps reinforced by perseveration. Of course, the topographically determined coincidence of the two syndromes implies their interpenetration. Also, amnestic factors, resulting from the same localization, may have a disturbing effect. This is due to an absence of the pertinent word in the formulation, which is thus retarded and requires modification (Lotmar).

Some general comments and interpretations might be added here concerning the localization of the various types of agrammatism. With regard to the expressive forms, it should not be thought that the grammatical knowledge or the feeling for the language is localized to a precise area. The relationship is rather to be explained in terms of functional impairment in those regions corresponding to stages in verbalization in which the syntactical and especially the grammatical processes are applied and so serve to match what is to be said to the thought pattern. It should be emphasized that the preexisting sentence pattern is decisive in word order, while in grammaticization the processes are applied to the words as they emerge. Similarly but with modification according to the course of the process, this also applied to sensory agrammatism. This, together with the fact that agrammatism is often secondary in nature, makes it clear that lesion and locus of function need not coincide. At least, this appears to be the case with regard to large lesions with their abundance of secondary phenomena.

Beyond the frontal or temporal localization, little can be said with certainty. For motor agrammatism as a secondary phenomenon, Broca's area is of causal significance. With regard to temporal paragrammatism, it is often obscured by severe paraphasia with lesion of Wernicke's area. It most likely has a functional correlation with the second and third temporal convolutions, for as the paraphasia diminishes, it may be clinically observed that both grammaticization and selection of words are closely related. This is also in agreement with occasional findings at autopsy. The coincidence of paragrammatism and sensory agrammatism suggests also that identical processes and/or substrata are involved in the origin of their symptoms. The localization of these disorders in the left T1 and T2 (even with localization elsewhere, the same mechanisms may be involved) suggests involvement in the acoustic portion of inner speech, in its participation in processes underlying the *grammaticization of speech;* also, there may be involvement of those higher psychic processes which are obstructed at the stage of their intervention in grammaticization.

Naturally, in this "localization" of agrammatism, the same reservations expressed in the discussion of "centers" must be taken into account.

It would be premature to attempt to fully explain the various forms in this manner. Little is known of the linguistic-psychological basis, and perhaps it is not yet possible to even approach these questions.

As a suggestion concerning these factors, it might be pointed out that the occurrence of certain small parts of speech, such as but, because, nevertheless, depends on an emotional state. Thus, we should investigate why these words are lacking, or their effect on sentence formation does not occur.

While these considerations must remain cautious, they nevertheless provide a starting point for further research on this central problem of aphasia theory.

If we consider these forms of expressive agrammatism from the functional and localizational points of view, we may see the following sequence: paragrammatism as the first in the sequence of processes subsequent to word choice; defective grammaticization of words; absence of such grammaticization; and, depending on the degree of speech difficulty, telegrammatism or Negersprache. After this comes linguistic puerilism as a still higher degree of linguistic poverty, impairment of the phonological side of speech (apparently occurring regularly with involvement of grammaticization). Clearly, this interpretation is in harmony with what we know of the localization of the temporal and frontal forms, as well as the similar effects upon these mechanisms emanating from higher psychic centers.

Sensory (impressive) agrammatism is discussed under the heading of word deafness.

Chapter 15

WORD DEAFNESS AND SPEECH DEAFNESS

WE NOW PROCEED to a discussion of the disorders affecting the *path from speech to thought*. It should again be emphasized, since it is important in the appraisal of the course of these disorders, including their anatomical outcome, that the later acquired sounds in school do not regularly correspond to the actual phonemes. Moreover, the sound of the word is comprehended as a whole and not as composed of letters and syllables (this is important in the evaluation of methods of examination often practiced!), nor do phonetic sound groups coincide with syllables. Accordingly, even in normals, by the law of economy, individual phonemes and sound groups are important in auditory comprehension insofar as is necessary to avoid misunderstanding. (Note the often adequate understanding of speech which is severely distorted by dysarthria.)

It follows from this that there is no special localization for the sounds of letters and syllables, much less for their parts. With regard to disturbances at sequential stages in the total process, it should be noted that in normals, particularly with stereotypic expressions and sentences, the entire series is not regularly traversed. In pathological cases, under the influence of the different assumed compensatory functions, this is even more marked. Here we are dealing with a schematic classification derived mainly from clinical phenomena and not from the nature of the disorders themselves, since our conclusions are indirect and concern only the area of understanding of word sounds. Regarding pathology, we must rely entirely on "conditions" and are quite in the dark as to components, especially since the most important evidence, that of self-inspection, is only rarely available.

Finally, it should be emphasized that the auxiliary words and other isolated words, except for those serving as one-word sentences, have no meaning in themselves. The common method of testing word-sound comprehension by repetition gives reliable results only when the latter is intact. For this reason, one should be cautious about drawing conclusions on the nature of these disorders, especially those appearing in repetition.

Disturbances in the processes underlying speech comprehension are grouped under the obviously inappropriate but established term of "word deafness" (Kussmaul). A description of this disorder accords with that of normals, since the latter has its basis partly in the pathological.

The most severe of these disorders is *unresponsiveness to spoken language* (Heilbronner). This occurs in the presence of intact awareness and adequate hearing, often combined with general acoustic unresponsiveness. The patient is unresponsive to the most intense acoustic stimuli and in this way is unlike other patients who react strongly to very slight impressions.

It has been observed that this unresponsiveness, even with structurally similar lesions, may be continuous or more often intermittent. However, through no discernible cause except for reinforcement by an attentional focus, unresponsiveness may alternate with periods of normal reaction. This indicates that functional factors may at times play a decisive role. This corresponds to the development of phenomenal structures upon the acoustic impression which differentiates out of the indifferent acoustic background. This finds support in the fact that along with unresponsiveness to language, there is perception of minute acoustic impressions, which refutes the assumption of destruction of discrete elements. If we conclude by analogy with normals and from occasional patient reports that this concerns the effect of attention, which from our hypothesis corresponds to processes mediated by centrifugal fibers in the sensory pathways, we may attribute the differences in behavior to differences in these processes. In the distribution of attention during conversation, a patient may be so fixed on his own speech that he does not notice what is said by other persons. This is supported by the fact that this acoustic structure is formed in the child under the influence of emotion. The importance of this emotional attitude is shown by the significance recently attributed to it in the analysis of normal perception (Klemm, 1921).

In other cases, this applies with persistence of the phenomena in spite of focusing on speech and the occurrence of acoustic hyperesthesia with simultaneous auditory hallucinations. In still other cases, lowered reactiveness of the perceptive elements may be involved. This interpretation is supported by similar observations on children with deficient ability to select auditory impressions out of the acoustic background (Froschels, 1918).

However, this does not explain continuous unresponsiveness. As there are few observations, it is uncertain whether a gradual habitual state involving different factors (inadequate initial function, increasing lack of interest) may not have developed. Consistent with this interpretation is the fact that patients affected to a slightly milder degree give a surprisingly uniform description of their acoustic perceptions; the importance of interest is demonstrated by a patient's recognition of the noise of a *specific* car.

Regarding localization, the phenomenon occurs with both unilateral and bilateral lesion of Wernicke's zone. The extent to which functional involvement of the acoustic center in Heschl's gyrus comes into play in an open question.

The discussion of centrifugal influences leads to the possibility of more peripheral effects, such as sensitization of the terminal organs. It may be difficult to distinguish these effects from impaired hearing.

The next stage, which combines several processes, embraces the *disorders of sound perception* and of *the understanding of word sounds*. This can be determined in only a few cases, since only the patients can provide information as to how and what they hear, and they are usually prevented from doing so by the accompanying disorders.

Formerly, it was assumed that patients heard what was spoken merely as noise or as a foreign language. The error of this view is shown by the variety of the phenomena, and by inference, the underlying processes. Sometimes, patients speak of noises, as in the loud talking of a crowd, in describing their sound perceptions. They constantly hear "drub-arub" or "toterotot." They may distinguish language from other sounds, or even hear the separate words, or distinguish vowels from consonants, though without perceiving them properly. Intonation may be correctly perceived in the absence of sound comprehension (as in threats, curses, challenges). Similarly, male and female voices and voices differing in other ways are distinguished even at a distance. Patients may be able to distinguish foreign languages and distinguish nonsense from their own language which is not understood. They may describe what is not understood as a foreign language, confuse different languages, recognize what they do not understand as having previously been uttered, even detect slight differences between words that they do not understand. Accordingly, patients often realize they are being addressed, are attentive, and notice their deficiency.

A proper understanding of these disorders must begin with characteristics of the auditory phenomena of colloquial language of which, unfortunately, we know little. Apart from our deficient knowledge of the relevant physiological processes, further difficulty lies in the fact that two adjuncts to the understanding of pathological phenomena, self-inspection and the inferences as to pathological processes to which it leads, will be lacking here, since these disorders are so often associated with disturbances of expressive speech (paraphasia). Contrary to the general view that the sensory material is principally affected, it is not so much peripheral, albeit intracerebral, pathological conditions that are most important. Rather, the main factor is in the sphere of the perception of acoustic tone patterns. Almost nothing can be said even about the grossest of these processes and their locus. Nor is it unlikely that processes within the realm of ordinary hearing may play a part. This is supported by observations in visual agnosia and also by the similarity with hearing disorders *sensu stricto,* such that demonstrated cases of peripheral hearing impairment have been taken as a starting point for the present subject (Armand). Moreover, the clinical picture of so-called subcortical sensory aphasia (pure word-deafness), which falls into this category, has vaguely defined boundaries with cerebral and labyrinthine disorders. Even with proof of a cerebral lesion, these boundaries cannot be drawn with confidence, with reference to the above differentiation.

The rarity of pertinent cases explains the poverty of precise observations, but these still suffice to show that within a specific range the disorders cause predictable rather than random effects. Balassa claims to have recently observed loss of tone quality in a single case. Besides the lowering of individual factors, defects of binaural hearing, of acoustic accomodation, even after-imagery and contrast phenomena may play a part. Clearly, we can hope for a real understanding of disorders of sound comprehension only when the acoustical impressions are as well known as the visual in regard to their "phenomenological types." In view of the scanty clinical data, any attempt at a detailed anatomical explanation appears premature and thoroughly speculative, especially as we know so little of the anatomical correlates of the stratification of comprehension. However, a few points of general importance may be considered.

The importance of the *situation* for comprehension of word sounds is evident in the influence of the *attunement* of that which follows the first word. The influence of the situation on word comprehension is clear without further explanation. It should be noted that the extent of the reaction varies without detectable cause. What was previously said concerning the difference between sounds, syllables, and words accounts for the fact that words are generally better comprehended than their sound components. Recognition of what is said as belonging to a foreign language is chiefly due to *musical factors* inherent in that language, just as its recognition as speech depends on the *speech melody*, which differentiates speech from other noises. *Accentuation* may explain why questions and threats, though not understood, are recognized to their meaning. In the recognition of different voices the *resonance of the acoustic phenomena* is decisive. The occasional recognition of vowels as such is unexplained (formants?). We may mention that similarities of sound will interfere in this process. The occasional deleterious effect of an individual or foreign manner of speaking suggests that the *word patterns* (Wortschema) abstracted from individual word images have lost some of their power to evoke a response. It is obvious that neither loss of word sounds nor disorder of conduction occurs, as has been generally alleged in explanation of the phenomena. The *feeling of familiarity* may be due to a single factor or several factors involved in the course of sound perception (familiar language, language of a familiar speaker, and so on). It is not known to what extent the *distribution of attention,* which normally has a marked effect on gestalt perception, comes into play. The *influence of emotional factors,* physical and psychic in nature, has been established. Something will be said later about the recognition of one's own deficiency.

Comprehension of word meaning presupposes adequate perception of word sounds or at least partial perception, since the understanding of garbled words, as in normals, indicates that the perceived word can be completed on the basis of partial perception.

The relation between the two is therefore varied. What is correctly perceived as to sound is also correctly understood, as long as the disorder does not affect higher levels. But understanding may also be lacking, as when words heard correctly as such are not perceived as accustomed structural patterns. Occasionally, one is surprised to find correct comprehension of the meaning of words when the understanding of word sounds is still markedly impaired. Usually the patient's own name is best retained, then simple words and numbers; shorter and more familiar words are better retained than those which are longer or less commonly used. At times, several repetitions are required for comprehension. Similarities of sound may lead to misunderstanding. The perceived word sound evokes a word belonging to the same category (eyes, ears—Bergson's "dynamic schema," Messer's "sphere awareness"), (Messer, 1906; Bergson, 1896; Delbruck, 1887), consistent with the fact that awareness of the proper category plays an outstanding part in the awareness of meaning. Along with this is the observation that the patient does not yet understand the names of objects, but does understand objects described. In polyglots, comprehension of the mother tongue generally outlasts comprehension of later learned languages. Difficulty in following the conversation of third parties is sometimes observed as a residual phenomenon. Consideration of superior word comprehension when presented in the context of a sentence leads us to the *comprehension of sentence meaning,* in which connection we shall also discuss the disorders of understanding dependent upon the dignity of various words. In comprehension, as in speech, sentence meaning has priority and the comprehension of names is secondary. Basic to this disorder is the failure to mobilize the word meaning from word sounds, which are otherwise adequately comprehended. The awareness of relationships, the structure of word-meaning concepts or conceptless meaning-awareness is disordered. Although we know very little about the factors which act in this complex process, we can reject the older assumption of an attenuation of the mnemonic availability of words. The role played by the "memory images" or more correctly the stimulation of the bases of memory is still quite obscure. It can only be said that it is impaired because of defective sensory structures due to the disorder, especially as these structures are not put together piecemeal.

The *preconstruction* is initiated by that which is initially heard and probably figures in the disturbance of synthetic comprehension. This is supported by the fact that occasionally only the last words are understood. In rapid speech, comprehension is probably impaired by rapid disappearance of the word sounds as a manifestation of reduced function. The complexity of the involved factors is illustrated by the occasional poorer comprehension of names for the parts of the body, even the simpler and more familiar ones, than comprehension of words in general. Here, as elsewhere, the sphere consciousness mentioned above comes into play. The involvement of concepts for things and concepts of words which are not acoustical components of inner speech explains that part of the phenomena noted in the *aids* toward word-meaning comprehension. Among these are the *motor attunement on perceived sounds,* often occurring spontaneously and derived from the infantile speech reflex (repetition in a low voice to aid deficient comprehension and, occasionally, writing motions as well) and, in turn, its reinforcement by seeing the corresponding object. In these "aids" we have to do with the preparation of the acoustic residues and/or their corresponding processes by other centripetal stimulations. *Speech melody* may be involved in the recognition of different voices and languages. The function of these aids has to do with the *concentration of attention on the meaning.* This suggests that the disorder results in an excessive attunement of attention on word sounds, and that in the background there is a curtailment of the span of awareness in general. The importance of *emotions* for the comprehension of words which correspond to them should also be mentioned. If the significance of the *situation* (the emotion is also a part of the psychic situation) acts either as a disturbing or supporting factor, this appears more clearly in failure of preexisting comprehension when the situation (or the subject of conversation) unexpectedly changes; this may also explain the varying behavior of these disorders. The impaired comprehension of the situation indicates how *defects of the higher psychic processes* can complicate those processes under discussion. The important contribution of the *musical elements* explains the importance of their absence or deficiency. We must also exclude lip-reading, which is quickly learned by some patients. The obvious functional gradation of these disorders negates an interpretation based upon destruction of specific elements of centers and supports the involvement of various disorders of processes underlying word comprehension. However, these cannot be localized in a word meaning center, since the meaning of the sentence is not the sum of the meanings of the individual words. In addition, testing with isolated words represents a thoroughly unnatural method, which is bound to fail especially in the case of auxiliary and grammatical words, which are altogether lacking in an isolated sense of their own. These lack the "denominative function" that is in the foreground of interest.

The comprehension of sentence meaning is often better than the comprehension of words. This is especially so with short sentences and does not always apply to longer ones, particularly when abstract material is concerned. Rapid speech may also have a disturbing effect. In the former, apart from the simpler comprehension of familiar turns of expression, the feeling for the language is obviously an aid (as a reflection of patterns acquired in learning to speak, in this case for sentences), since rearranging the sentence facilitates understanding. Instructions of any complexity are carried out slowly or not at all, because words understood separately may not be understood in context, unless the context is quite unambiguous. Longer sentences are understood only when broken up into shorter ones.

The understanding of these two forms is furthered by a knowledge of the representation of relationships both through word order (syntax) and grammaticization *sensu stricto*. While in the first instance, comprehension of word order is disturbed (we may speak of *impressive asyntaxia*), disorders of the second type concern what is called *sensory (impressive) agrammatism* (in the narrow sense). Disturbance of stages in the comprehension of sentence meaning which correspond to the grammaticization of the sentence, insofar as both characterize relationships, will disturb to a varying extent the comprehension of these relationships. There may also be a loss of knowledge of sentence form or of its accompanying language feeling (Sprachgefühl). The latter also appears as an inability to form a meaningful sentence from available words in spite of correct thought formulation. On the impressive side, it appears as a lack of comprehension of the purpose of the whole in spite of comprehension of the individual words; the linguistic pattern which underlies the statement is not understood. These phenomena were first clearly understood and systematically studied by E. Salomon.

As pointed out in the introductory remarks on agrammatism, this latter form is generally not separated from the others, both for clinical considerations (e.g. the coexistence of expressive and sensory agrammatism) as well as psychological considerations (e.g. the same process is at one time centrifugal and at another centripetal). However, this disorder does belong with the defects of comprehension of sentence meaning, a fact which suggests that sensory agrammatism should be treated more fully within the category of word-deafness.

This includes cases in which the meaning of prepositions or other auxiliary words uttered in speech is either confused or not understood. It also includes grammatical incomprehension, in which the word sounds are adequately comprehended but not the inflections or similar grammatical modifications of the words, so that the sentence meaning is misunderstood or is not understood at all. (Of course, deficient auditory perception may also hinder the more difficult acoustic embodiment of a grammatical formulation.) A distinction should be made between lack of comprehension of the grammatical forms of correct speech and inadequate recognition of incorrect forms. In the former, the listener lacks the feeling, based on early acquired analogies, for the grammatical structures of linguistic devices employed by the speaker. The thought pattern customarily associated with this grammatical structure cannot be developed. The patient does not understand the sentence because he has not grasped the fundamental relationships corresponding to the thought pattern, in spite of the fact that the individual words are understood. In this regard, we should mention some differences which arise if linguistic comprehension first seizes object-naming or syntax. Less severe disorders entail uncertainty and hesitation of comprehension in which the retained understanding of intonational pattern will have a helpful effect. This is not so for incorrect grammatical material used in testing. Here, the feeling for the language (the knowledge gained in school recedes far into the background) acts on the basis of automatized analogies. In pathological cases, it either does not act or does so inadequately, so that the process does not lead to the proper correction. Accordingly, this has nothing to do with sequence formation of a motor type.

In the evaluation of these cases, one must keep in mind the following: a patient who is by no means demented and who correctly performs complex commands will calmly accept such sentences as "der Bäcker wird gebacken" (the baker is going to be baked) or "der Hund führt den Herrn an der Leine (the dog leads the master on the leash).* He may recognize the incorrect construction only after several questions and hints. This is because in economical fashion (even in normals) we take in only as much of the words forming the sentence as necessary to derive its meaning. This is assumed for every utterance which is derived from a knowledge of things and their relationships. This is best illustrated by such a sentence as "Missionar Wilder fressen" ('missionaries eat savages' or 'savages eat missionaries'),† where although the possibility of misunderstanding exists formally, there will be no doubt as to the meaning. The patient has often correctly understood such sentences, and only in expression is he unable to give them proper form. (Cf. also the facts of sign language and the language of deaf-mutes.) The sense of the reversible sentence is so unambiguous and compelling (logical irreversibility!) that the possibility of a reversal does not enter the patient's mind.

Preconstruction has been discussed in the description of normal language to explain sentence comprehension. This applies to both grammaticization of words and the word order. Inaudible *simultaneous speech* is common and is of consequence to the extent that when defective it will also disturb the preconstruction, necessitating

---

Editor's Note: The examples are not very telling in English. In German either subject or object comes before the verb, so that the expression is ambiguous unless one is in the masculine singular, where there is a formal difference between nominative and accusative cases. The first example does not seem convincing even in German; the author may have been thinking of "das Brot bäckt den Bächer" (the bread bakes the baker) which could be understood by the patient as "das Brot bäckt der Bächer" (bread is baked by the Baker), but he has put it into a form where the illogicality is as conspicuous in German as in English.

†The sentence "Missionare fressen Wilder" is misprinted in the source as Missionar Wilder fressen, which is unnatural German.

corrections just as in speech. Correct comprehension of the *musical elements* (sentence melody, accent) as proved by nonecholalic repetition in the presence of a loss of speech comprehension, show that the avaliability of "residua" in addition to factors of a purely perceptual nature plays a part.

In addition to these disorders, there are others outside the field of pathological speech comprehension, namely the *intellectual functions* connected with sentence comprehension, to which a bridge is provided by the understanding of the abstract. Thus, in recovery, the patient comes to recognize the meaninglessness of nonsense sentences. This relates to the mental processes underlying predication and is beyond the scope of our present discussion. The patient lacks understanding of words in a figurative sense, of formulae, proverbs, puns and jokes. It is basic to this disorder that sentence comprehension becomes worse when two or more smaller sentences, separately comprehensible, are brought into relation (cf. "thought interrelationships"; Bühler, 1908). Sometimes the understanding of other "semantic functions" (Head) is also lacking (whether separately is doubtful), such as that for the position of hands on the clock; but this may be preserved in isolation in the presence of other severe disorders.

Other factors in addition to these come into consideration. The detection and evaluation of these is complicated by the lack of typical forms of disorder which can support conclusions as to their nature. There are also compensatory "makeshifts" of the cerebral apparatus which hinder the delineation of the disruptive factors. We must confine our discussion to the causative factors, especially as it is always several that are involved. One important factor is the difficulty, at times primary and at times due to deficient comprehension of sentence meaning, in the feeling for the situation, the importance of which for speech and comprehension has already been discussed. (The contribution of accompanying gesture and mimicry needs only to be mentioned.) In addition, especially in the case of long sentences, there is reduced memory capacity and consequent difficulty in following the line of thought as well as defective auditory preconstruction and inability to comprehend the "resultant" word meaning. Diminished auditory retention (especially in the case of rapid speech) has a similar effect, as well as the frequently reduced span of awareness in the aphasic. Lastly, there is the important factor of proper distribution of attention (e.g. directing the attention to word sounds with serious impairment of the comprehension of word-meaning). The same factor is involved, though not in sentence comprehension, when the patient is more involved with the object than with the action with which it is to be performed. Head emphasized the additional difficulty in comprehension of sentence meaning when a choice among several possibilities is required, a fact partly related to the above.

From the discussion, we may infer that the basic pathological tendency lies in the *disordered combination of perceived acoustic sequences into a whole*. We may contrast this with disordered word-sound comprehension, in which there is an inability to combine the meaning of the sentence by way of words only partially understood.

The abbreviated processes of comprehension in normals are also noted in pathological cases, especially when practiced expressions lead to the corresponding action almost by reflex (e.g. "a car!"—jumping aside).

The presence or absence of *understanding of one's own deficiency* is usually of decisive importance; it will vary and will necessitate different explanations according to its form. In unresponsiveness we can see that the attunement of attention is important. In cases of partial understanding of words and sentences, the comprehension that is achieved will conceal the partial deficiency. The statements of patients must be carefully checked, because they will often confuse impairments of comprehension with those of hearing.

In this regard, we must account for the usually rapid *restitution* of the defective processes underlying auditory perception and what this implies (in the clinical sense) of the greater facility of these processes. We may say that, especially in the above impressive process, volition and its accompaniments and that which has to do with practice in those expressive processes toward which it leads (cf. what was said earlier concerning the effect of practice) is either lacking or present outside of awareness.

In conclusion, we must mention the *mild word deafness usually observed in cases of motor aphasia*. In acute cases, this can be explained by the neighboring effects of the frontal lesion and secondarily by the possibility of total aphasia with a sensory component usually of short duration. Another important factor is probably the narrowing of awareness and need for repetition, which is also disordered and therefore insufficient for this purpose, for the understanding of longer sentences.

We summarized the processes activated in speech comprehension as serving for conduction of the serially perceived multitude of auditory impressions and their transformation into meaningful thoughts. These functions, by their limitation to the set of conventional phonemes utilized in meaningful discourse, are organized into a sphere to which auditory sensation is subordinated, with separate localization of its anatomophysiological mechanisms. It follows that the assumption of separate centers for letters, syllables and words, and of the memory images of these entities supposedly stored in such centers is unconvincing.

The localization of these mechanisms concerns the central and, in part, the posterior portion of the superior temporal convolution, first studied by Wernicke, just anterior to the acoustic center in the (Heschl's) transverse convolution. The part of that convolution just anterior is important for the musical component. Regarding processes of conductance to the psychic mechanisms, we may assume for the latter an "expanded Wernicke's zone," the location of which is not known. We also know little of the extent of participation of the right temporal lobe in functions carried out beyond the acoustic center and commonly attributed to the left Wernicke center. This also complicates the interpretation of the details of these disorders.

In this discussion, we have mentioned the *complication with true hearing disorders* of peripheral and central origin. With respect to the latter, this is readily understood from what has just been said. As to differential diagnosis, symptoms pertaining to peripheral hearing impairment must be considered, as well as the expressive disorders often accompanying central defects of speech comprehension. The latter are especially involved in the rare syndrome of isolated pure ("subcortical") sensory aphasia, where only auditory perception is impaired. For a time it was held that intactness of the so-called Bezold's auditory scale from b1 to g2 guaranteed comprehension. This is incorrect as the scale may be preserved in severe cases of word-deafness.

An *isolated sound-deafness* has recently been observed and held to relate to a circumscribed localization (in T3 and OT; Kehrer, 1913; Henschen, 1917; Goldstein, 1923). Aside from clinico-anatomical objections, we must consider the fact that spoken words are among the noises. Also, the speech melody and other musical elements of speech form a bridge between speech and music. This speaks against the localization of the three functions in different parts of the cerebral cortex.

Chapter 16

ALEXIA

THE TERM word-blindness, or alexia, comprises various disorders affecting visual perception and the comprehension of writing and its meaningful units (words and sentences), in which defects of visual acuity and the visual field play no part. Although alexia is one form of visual agnosia, as concerns comprehension of the meaning of larger units, it exceeds the bounds of visual agnosia into the sphere of thinking.

On casual inspection, the phenomena of alexia fall into two categories, as in the case of word-deafness. Depending on whether primary or secondary identification is involved, there is either a disorder of the perception of the word form or of the word meaning. On closer investigation, not only do we see again the primacy of the sentence as the bearer of the whole meaning but also a number of other processes, disorders of which lead to a variety of phenomena. As in auditory perception, where it is not the entire letter content that is involved but only the most characteristic elements, the perception of word form does not always require all the letters in the word.

In the most severe of these disorders there is a kind of unresponsiveness in which a printed sheet given to a patient will not even be turned to its proper position. This nonrecognition of the printed page and the total lack of recognition of letters or even of the patient's own signature, otherwise practically always recognized, forms a transition to visual agnosia. Other patients recognize letters (and figures) as such, but confuse them with each other or with notes or other numerals. Figures similar to letters are recognized, then a few letters, perhaps only the small ones, or the patient's own well-practiced initials; this may be especially so for simple letters (occasionally by recognition of the characteristic part of the letter), at times without ability to provide their names. Familiar handwriting is differentiated from other writing. Diphthongs and consonants are often harder to recognize; then short words, which are read correctly in the face of poor reading of the constituent letters; words of similar morphology are confused, and longer words are read only by spelling or not at all. These differences between the comprehension of words and letters have led to the terms *literal* and *verbal alexia*. In evaluating these forms, the artificiality of testing for the former plays a part, as well as the neglect of the fact of perception of the gestalt of a word, e.g. at times long words are read better than shorter ones. Differences in legibility according to type and familiarity and between printing and handwriting also have an influence. Patients may be unable to read formulae (compounds and the like), while certain letters otherwise not read, when combined into a symbol, a business form, or the like, may be read correctly and with comprehension. Reading aloud may help with comprehension, occasionally requiring several repetitions. Sometimes patients must recite the alphabet to recognize letters presented them. When words read are not understood, reading aloud does not evoke their meaning. Reading through spelling may help with longer words which are not recognized as a whole, as in normals, or with shorter ones. Commonly, reading aloud adds to the difficulty, as an additional effort, and especially because of greater fixation of attention by the new motor act. This consideration explains the occasional differences between reading aloud and silent reading. (The corresponding movements may be performed with the head or masked in eye movements, even without a model.) Some patients may recognize only that which they write and are otherwise unable to read. This applies only to written material, since printed matter was previously never copied in the same form. However, these aids fail in patients who have read little. Visual aids—objects displayed, pictures, colors—also help in reading comprehension. These *aids* often develop rapidly and are designed to conceal the disorder. With improvement, the words are completed by completion of elements partially read. Sometimes the disorder affects only a certain kind of writing, shorthand, or only a certain language, in both instances generally acquired late (Ribot's rule). In such cases, letters of the lost language which occur in the retained language are read in the latter (this is evidence against the assumption of fixed engrams and supports the gestalt quality). At times, all languages suffer alike. The accentuation of words that are not understood is often incorrect, or both accentuation and rythm, because they are determined by the context, often appear late and thus disturb the comprehension of meaning which is dependent on them. But the whole sentence may also be read with proper accent and intonation and still without comprehension, evidently because these factors are established by practice. Disorders of reading at this stage concern the meaning of recognized single words, but still also disturb the meaningful comprehension of the sentence in various ways, and lead the patient to guess at the sentence meaning; this is consistent with the fact that there may be disturbance of comprehension of semantically opposite sentences formulated of the same words. The basis of these disorders corresponds to that of defects of auditory comprehension. The *duration of the disorder* may be permanent, while its intensity often exhibits some fluctuation. Slight disorders undetectable by ordinary testing will sometimes be revealed by tachistoscopic examination by prolonged reaction times. A disorder corresponding to impressive agrammatism also occurs here. In *differential diagnosis,* reading disorders due to restriction of the visual field, especially the right, may interfere with forward gaze necessary for reading. These must be taken into consideration, as well as a reading defect appearing in skips, and the loss of one's place, said to be due to irregular defects in the eye movements which accompany reading (Poppelreuter, 1917).

We should mention the "dyslexia" or "reading shyness" (Lesescheu) first described by Berlin, which consists (in paresis or arteriosclerotic brain damage) of initial correct reading with rapid, painful and recurrent fatigue. This phenomenon may be analogous to dysbasia angiosclerotica (intermittent claudication) in the corresponding region of the brain (Pick, 1891).

Mention should also be made of *paralexia due to speech disorder,* which might be better termed "paraphasic reading." Everything said of paraphasia holds true here as well, in addition to inferences from slips of the tongue in normals (or from mistakes in reading). If the defective reading is not due to defective word comprehension (by evidence other than writing) which is often itself disordered (pointing, rephrasing the word!), the tempo (usually rapid in paraphasia and paragraphia) and other accompanying symptoms will permit a differential diagnosis. Paraphasic reading may also impair reading comprehension because the "mispronounced" word, especially if actually or seemingly important, is misheard and thereby alters the meaning given it in reading.

By *congenital* (familial) *word blindness* (Righetti, 1900; Peters, 1908; Brissaud, 1904; Hinshelwood, 1900; Plate, 1909; Fildes, 1921) or reading difficulty is meant a disorder occurring not only with other intellectual defects but also independently in children of high intelligence. It consists of inability to read or difficulty in reading, even to understand the meaning of very short words. Writing is more successful.

We should begin our *description of alexia* by remarking that it involves a disorder of a specialized function, which because it is acquired late is more vulnerable. The written (or printed) word is a symbol for speech, acoustic or thought symbols. For this reason, reading is dependent not only on normal visual perception and its subsequent processing but also to some extent on the sparing of those functions serving the speech symbols and associations. In view of the combined visual-acoustic-motor function which is acquired in learning to read and still used by less skillful readers, we shall have to distinguish between the *primarily visually determined disorders* and those in which components affected extraneously *secondarily* impair the combinatory function. Thus, motor or acoustic-sensory aphasic disorders may also indirectly affect reading. The skillful reader, who can read with comprehension without the above, suffers less than one who reads through spelling and reading aloud.

The unity of word and sentence is to be emphasized as important for all forms of disorder. The importance of the word as a unit stands in contrast to its synthesis from letters and syllables in school, which is linguistically and physiologically unjustified. Careful consideration must also be given to the influence of general factors. Formerly, it was assumed (Grashey, 1884; Goldscheider and Müller, 1893) that reading was accomplished by spelling and for this reason would be damaged by lowered memory capacity, through forgetting the letters just read. However, in addition to the lack of evidence of lowered memory capacity and the fact that for the most part reading occurs differently (succession and chiefly simultaneity), other factors have been estab-

(succession and chiefly simultaneously), other factors have been established as the cause of alexia. Of course, disorders of perception and memory certainly are important here, as well as in the visual comprehension of the forms and their meaning. Moreover, they are important in sentence comprehension, which again is not a summation of the meanings of individual words. In sentence production, a "preconstruction" from what has already been read participates, which if disordered damages the whole. Both are bound to suffer from the increased reading difficulty, since attention is diverted from its goal, the meaning of what is read, and is fixed mainly on the visual or motor element. This is even more true in cases of spelling difficulty, where attention must be directed not to the word as a whole but to the individual letters and their motor production. These different factors—poor overall grasp due to insufficient discrete attention, poor distribution of attention, and narrowness of the span of awareness—must await a special empirical analysis. It should be noted that for alexia in polyglots, Ribot's rule holds (with some exceptions). According to the accounts of patients, we can infer a loss of visual images of letters and words, at times with competely retained object images. Saloz, the aphasic physician, spoke of the "fading away of the inwardly seen letters" (by means of which the agraphic patient often writes). Occasionally, there is correct perception of written forms, confirmed by digit recognition, which rules out a primary disorder of form perception. This suggests, in relation to disorder of the visual image, that one form of alexia is determined by the nonrecognition of correctly perceived written forms. In other cases, the disorder affects form perception, only the simplest forms, crudest outlines, or parts of letters being perceived (letters appearing slanted or inverted.) From other accounts, we can infer a defect of directional concepts, as well as in the discrimination of directional differences. We may infer from the erroneous reactions of many patients the presence of visual shifts and compression, suggesting the loss of the perception of the visual gestalt as a coherent entity. Words and sentences are no longer perceived as familiar structural entities and for this reason are perceived incorrectly. The variety of these disorders probably explains why some patients correctly perceive a whole word while unable to perceive the constituent letters. Practice and filling-in are important as well as certain outlines produced by the letter combinations which may extend above or below the line and by the narrowed attentional field. If the perception of the word as a whole represents the norm, the contrary, namely better reading of individual letters, may be due to the strong and persistent influence of schooling. This is supported by the order of recovery. First, it is possible to read figures, then words, and finally letters. The importance of the gestalt also appears in the fact that patients are at times unable to find letters in words, which are otherwise recognized in isolation. In milder cases, confusions due to similar form certainly play a part.

The common disparity of better recognition of written than printed material is readily understandable (more practice). But the contrary also occurs. This difference in the patient's behavior toward digits and letters is not inconsistent with the hypothesis of gestalt perception, since we consider not only the gestalt as such but also its degree of facility from practice (the letter gestalt is acquired later and only by artificial separation; the figure gestalt is stable from the beginning and linguistically older).

In favor of the gestalt theory is the fact that in Japan, Chinese ideographic characters (ed. kangi) are more resistant to disorder than the Japanese characters (ed. kana), evidently because of their pictorial quality (Asayama, 1914). In cases where letters are not recognized but can be distinguished from similar marks, familiarity may also play a part. If letter perception is intact, defective comprehension may occur from lack of correspondence with the word sound (phoneme), though satisfactory reproduction of the sound may occur even with a suboptimal total visual impression. We must also consider errors relating to the musical elements (sentence melody, accent) due to deficient visual perception. These aids from the sound-image of the word elicit the motoric speech and writing components of the inner word. These in turn act as aids in reading, as seen not only in the corresponding hand movements but occasionally in movements of the head as well. The benefit of soft pronounciation during reading, well known in normals, is especially common in such patients.

The effect of these aids may be summarized as follows: structural relationships established in the acquisition of reading as well as in the ancillary acquisition of writing, which represent the expanded "inner speech," reappear compulsively when the acquired attenuated process is lost or disordered. Their failure, especially word sound which is so indispensable to the unskilled reader, will have an intense effect on the phenomena, perhaps even on some phenomena individually. In other cases of severe word-blindness in which the visual and auditory components of the inner speech are retained, and where form perception of writing is intact, as demonstrated by correct copying, the defect lies in the impaired synchronization of functions which normally provide for the *understanding of writing*. This also includes patients who understand several words of what is read, but not the meaning of the entire sentence.

With regard to the influence of other aphasic disorders on reading comprehension, the speech defect of motor aphasia will disturb reading to different degrees. This especially affects reading through spelling, as in the less skillful reader, at least as concerns longer words, whereas short words which have been established as "gestalts" are unaffected. However, this interpretation is questionable with respect to reflex acoustic stimulation of this process. Moreover, there are many cases with intact reading in spite of damage to this component. Certainly, in acute cases the effects of diaschisis must be taken into account. Rarely, word-blindness may outlast the speech disorder (complication with similarly localized lesion?). As noted previously, foreign languages may be more severely impaired, and as the motor aphasia improves, reading also returns. It is evident that the retardation of reading, attentional focus on the obstructed act, even defects of memory must impair in reading the comprehension of sentence meaning. Occasional severe disorders of reading comprehension may be due to a strong motor-speech predisposition. The great importance of the word sound in reading appeared initially to justify the view taken from temporal lesion with speech-deafness that disordered reading was necessarily dependent on speech-deafness. However, it has been found that these reading disorders may be more intense than the word-deafness and may be occasioned by direct or indirect (proximity effect) involvement of the functional alexia zone (angular gyrus).

Since writing is the secondary association of a symbol with the heard or spoken word, any disorder of the sound image, no matter as to degree or origin, will impair reading just as a disorder in the relation between the written and audible word. The complexity of the task and the amount of practice in reading are especially important in determining the extent of the disorder. In so-called total aphasia, reading will be entirely lacking, the degree of its recovery depending on these conditions. *Alexia occurring with mind-blindness* (Seelenblindheit) is a secondary disorder. When an early symptom, it may only be due to proximity effects of the visual sphere or its afferent pathways. In permanent cases, it is to be explained by a lowered function of neuronal pools associated with the special visual speech structures. The minor influence of alexia on the functions of spoken language is in contrast to what has just been said and can be understood from the *secondary nature of writing*. The paraphasia which occasionally accompanies word-blindness is probably a complication or a diaschisis effect. Perseveration might also play a role in alexia, but a distinction must be made between the motor type (the most common) and that which affects visual functions. Patients with alexia ordinarily notice quite early the lack of comprehension. Sometimes, meaningless combinations of letters are read, seemingly with the feeling that the patient is truly reading, though there is prior or subsequent awareness of the disorder. The patient may attribute to his presumed reading trains of thoughts which are induced by the alexia, especially when accompanied by jargon aphasia. Similar considerations apply to the correctly perceived word image and sentence comprehension to which it leads, taking into account the functional and chronological differences between visual and auditory perception, as discussed with speech-deafness. As in that case, general functional phenomena are also of great importance. The often striking and irregular variation of these defects, even with regard to the same task, speaks against their interpretation as due to an absence of specific images or residua. The same mental processes take place in reading with comprehension, as concerns word and sentence meaning, as in auditory comprehension. Thus, analogous defects of syntactical and grammatical comprehension, i.e impressive agrammatism, will be found. The reader is referred to that section for a more extensive account. Uncertainties in the interpretation of inability to perform complex commands, emphasized in the previous section, are still more applicable in this case (memory). The evidence that in normal reading (Messmer, 1904) relational elements are *inferred* more from the grammatical feeling than from what is actually read makes it likely that a corresponding defect occurs in reading, especially with disorders of sentence comprehension. Since the grammatical feeling is just developing in the child, this may be of importance in the defect of so-called *congenital reading difficulty* and in infantile agrammatism. In evaluating the relevant data, one must not overlook the natural occurrence of substitute constructions. Congenital reading difficulty is due to a serious deficiency in the perception and retention of visual forms, commonly accompanied by a corresponding defect in the auditory sphere. In addition, there is difficulty in establishing a connection between symbols (letters) and names, as well as poor retention of words read. The discrepancy between correct letter perception and poor reading is explained mainly by defective gestalt perception, in which there may be a disorder of the grasp of the whole. From the anatomicophysiological point of view, this is probably a (hereditary) defect in development of regions concerned with reading and a consequent inability of the involved functions to develop.

In defining the concept of alexia, we emphasized the absence of any basic visual disorders. A sharp delimitation of processes of perception from those of sensation is not possible, especially in view of evidence from work on mind-blindness, and suggests caution regarding too severe a differentiation. This is in agreement with what has been said of defects in form perception, as well as the statements of certain patients that letters appear as if "smeared." This does not alter the account of alexia as a disorder of various functions which coordinate higher integrating functions, just as word-deafness is a disorder of the integrative functions of Wernicke's zone.

The *preference for the left hemisphere* also applies to alexia or for left-handed persons the right hemisphere. Rare cases have been described of so-called "crossed aphasia," in which the lesion responsible for the alexia was situated in the right hemisphere of right-handed patients.

Delineation of the respective contribution of the right and left hemisphere in the various processes is impossible for now. Even with retention of reading with partial bilateral destruction of the angular gyrus region, we cannot determine how much of that region must be intact to preserve function. It seems unlikely that the angular gyrus is coextensive with a homogeneously developed cortical field in view of the number of functions there united. The obviously stratified arrangement of the alexias suggests a corresponding classification of their physiological and anatomical substrata, but many cases studied both clinically and anatomically from this point of view would be required before it is possible to make a precise local diagnosis. Letters are (not always simple) forms which differ from other signs only by convention as visual symbols for certain phonemes, a relationship which explains the differentiation between the anatomicophysiological mechanisms associated with alexia from those associated with other visual form recognitions. This indicates how unconvincing is the notion of a "word reading center" (and, of course, all the more a "letter center") as loci of storage of the corresponding memory images. Complex hypotheses have been devised to account for the relation of literal alexia to mind-blindness (ed. visual agnosia), or nonrecognition of letters and good recognition of objects, without taking into account the fact that letter images *per se* have neither seperate existence nor meaning.

Although a more precise delimitation is not currently possible, the angular gyrus may be designated the locus of the neuronal pools which correspond to these processes, between the optic-motor and visual centers, Wernicke's area and the psychic regions.

In the white matter of this gyrus are located, in addition to the optic radiation, the pathways from the visual center to the gyrus, and those from it to the higher centers. These latter serve for comprehension, and it is tempting to suggest, apart from the frequent hemianopsia which is thus explained, an anatomical differentiation of the various forms of alexia (subcortical with intactness of the word image, i.e. pure alexia, and cortical with disorder of the word image and all of its consequences.) However, not only is this theoretically erroneous, but it has been found to be untenable on clinical and anatomical grounds. It has been shown repeatedly (Dejerine, Pötzl, Bonvicini) that pure alexia is found with superficial and deep lesion of the lingual and fusiform gyri.

Chapter 17

AGRAPHIA

AGRAPHIA CONCERNS those disorders which affect writing as a symbol for thought, in the presence of intact intelligence and free motility *sensu stricto*. Just as dysarthria was excluded from motor aphasia, agraphia excludes all those disorders (motor and sensory, including kinesthetic) which affect primarily the performance of the executive organ which are probable complications due to the proximity of the involved centers (foot of F2 and hand center). Thus, when we speak of "motor" agraphia we have in mind only those disorders with involvement of the center in F2 analogous to Broca's region, as distinguished from those which derive from damage to the visual center in the angular gyrus.

In severe cases in which the operation of the writing mechanism (as directly concerns praxis) is intact, the patient may write nothing at all or only his name, which is the most highly automatized performance, or similar formulae. Then the patient makes meaningless hooks, among which a letter or two may be recognizable; letters are omitted, interchanged, reduplicated; at times words can be written but not the individual letters. The patient commonly writes slowly with hesitation in fragments that are generally nonsensical and usually do not correspond to syllabic division. Sometimes, letter writing is good when writing otherwise is defective. The patient may write rapidly at times in order to sustain the happenstance of an automatized "writing melody." Here also belongs the contrast in difficulty of the writing of individual words to command compared to the facility with the same words in a sentence.

Rarely, writing with the right hand is impaired with preserved ability to copy. (cf. apraxia theory and our comments regarding deaf-mutes who develop an aphasia.) Sometimes the patient cannot event write to dictation using block letters.

In accordance with Ribot's rule, in polyglots the latest acquired

[111]

languages are generally most affected, sometimes in the presence of their correct speech. *Copying* is often no better than *spontaneous writing*, but sometimes is preserved without comprehension; occasionally, there is correct copying of printed material in longhand (ed. transliteration). Copying one's own name is sometimes worse than a spontaneous signature (contrast of volition and automatism). The copy may match the model in an obvious manner (ed. slavish copying) or may be independent of the model. Copying is certainly better than spontaneous writing and may be good in the face of complete agraphia. However, the reverse is occasionally true. Often short words can be copied smoothly, but longer words take more time, almost to the point of drawing from the model.

If the patient's retention of written matter is defective, removal of the model will lead to deterioration in performance with omission of letters and other errors. Contrary to the usual case, writing is sometimes better than speaking. Movements of the head and of the hand in the air (even passively), which helps in imitation, are effective as aids. Showing the patient the letters sometimes helps, as well as having the patient pronounce the words before writing them.

A special form of writing disorder is *paragraphia,* characterized by the occurrence, in patients without other defects of writing, of substitutions in writing which range, like paraphasia, from verbal and literal disturbances to jargon. Often the paragraphic word corresponds to the paraphasia pronounced, but sometimes the two diverge. The patient may pronounce words correctly and nonetheless write them incorrectly, or he may write down paraphasic utterances with less success. Perseveration is often found with paragraphia.

Disorders of orthography are a common accompaniment of the different forms of aphasia. Occasionally, they are the only residual after recovery from a temporal aphasia.

Obviously from what has been said of the secondary nature of written symbols, defective linguistic sentence construction (agrammatism) can occur with otherwise correct writing; this may be called "written agrammatism." However, according to the differences between speech and writing, it may be lacking in the latter or present in a mild form. The attitude of the patient toward his errors varies, occasionally such that the error is felt without the ability for it to be determined with certainty or corrected.

Our account of agraphic disorders will have to consider three fundamental factors: (1) The complexity of this function, writing being a late acquisition both culturally and individually and a symbol for the spoken or heard word, which in turn is a symbol for what is thought; (2) the excitation and execution of writing movements, even for the skilled writer, is not a simple motor act, their accomplishment bound to the corresponding motor centers; rather, as in the case of speech, writing is subject to a multitude of influences relayed from higher regions through an integrating center (not coordinating, in the motor sense) developed for this purpose. (3) The level of this function varies in the normal individual. This last factor accounts for the use or redevelopment of aids which are formed in learning to write and later more or less discarded. The first factor is decisive for the differentiation of agraphic disorders into those which develop with the conversion of speech symbols into written symbols, and those which appear as a part of the utilization of speech symbols as an expression of thought in which the written symbols are a secondary though necessary accompaniment.

In addition, there are *general disordered states,* disorders of attentional distribution, narrowed awareness, memory disorder, which may be more operative here than in other dysfunctions, since the functional series is longer and more complicated. It is impossible to discuss this theoretically in all its ramifications, nor is it possible in individual cases to clearly distinguish these from primary pathogenetic factors. In regard to attentional distribution, we must emphasize the normal direction of attention toward the meaning of what is to be written and the pathological concentration of attention more intensely on the writing. The disorder of chronological relationships which occurs in pathological states between thinking, speaking, and writing may also be important. This suggests again that the findings derived from learning experiments are significant.

A lowered capacity for observation which may develop at various stages of the process may also be important (omission of letters, defective sentence construction). In writing from dictation, there may be inability to remember the sentence. Perseveration is an important pathological factor, particularly in temporal lobe disturbances. If there is repetition of the same hooks and letters, the locus of the basic defect is likely to be in the motor area for writing. In repetition of the same words, it is presumably at a higher stage in the series of processes.

Fatigue also plays a part. It appears in the occurrence of paraphasias and perseverations in writing when these features are lacking (in the developing or recovery stage) in spoken language. This factor, which is effective in a quantitative manner, can be of significance diagnostically in cases of functionally determined defects (e.g. after epileptic attacks.) The concurrence of correct automatic writing with disordered volitional writing indicates that memory images are not involved in this condition.

In a certain sense, writing counteracts impairments in speech insofar as in writing, the model of what is to be written and the subsequent linguistic formulation which the model permits and indeed facilitates constitute a favorable factor.

The contrast between automatism and volition, important in the phenomenon of motor aphasia, also appears in writing but not as strongly; both conditions are to be appraised in an analogous manner.

Lastly, from the point of view of speech psychology, it must be remembered that the letter (as the presumed elemental unit) and the word do not stand in a mutual relationship of simple and more difficult. Instead, the relationship is quite variable, depending on attention to word pattern or the later acquired spelling.

In the multiplicity of these factors, the predisposition to or development of different *speech* (and *conceptual*) *types* may influence in some fashion the forms of the disturbance (more severe disorder in the visual type) (Pick, 1923).

According to the development of writing, two factors are of special importance in a consideration of agraphic defects: first, the image of the script, which is a leading factor in learning to write but is submerged in the accomplished writer; second, the arousal of the conditions necessary for writing, which even in a modestly experienced writer gradually become automatized motor structures (motion melodies). Similarly, the arousal process also becomes largely automatic and may originate anywhere, particularly from the psychic sphere.

The cortical functional region for the script image is that part of the angular gyrus discussed in relation to alexia. Presumably, as with Broca's area in motor aphasia, transfer (activated through various modes, from what is thought, heard, read) of the linguistically formulated, previously homogeneous thought into writing occurs. Processes take place in the region anterior to the hand center and superordinate to that center (foot of F2) which involve successive stimulation of corresponding sequences in the hand center.

The disorders will thus consist of those in which either the script image or its arousal fails, and those in which other component factors are defective, viz: childhood aids in learning to write, and in the patient, as well as fundamental factors in writing which these latter indirectly impair. Accordingly, the first group may be subdivided into a *visual* and *motor form* of *agraphia*. The other group contains those agraphic disorders which accompany symptoms of primary motor speech or sensory disturbance affecting speech comprehension. Since writing is expressed through secondary symbols, it cannot remain intact with disturbance of the immediately affected elements because of the intimate relationship of the various components of inner speech.

Although this differentiation appears clear theoretically, the relevant and diagnostically desirable factors have not been sufficiently clarified to know whether there is a disturbance of the coordination of the script images to the phonemes or of the relevant sequences of motion. Regarding disorders of the "writing melody," this is due to the relative rarity of anatomically verified and clinically pure cases (the clinical identification of this form is not yet as reliable as the others.) However, for all forms, it is generally due to the complexity of the phenomena, which is largely under the influence of early compensatory functions. It is clear that the whole situation remains in doubt from the contradictory interpretations which are presently given even to identical cases.

This is seen in the *relation between alexia and agraphia,* which appears so simple but is not a direct dependence (agraphia is not always a consequence of alexia!). Cases of intact writing with word-blindness may be interpreted by holding that the arousal of the motor structures has become independent, sometimes only for the trained right hand, but occasionally also for the obviously simultaneously trained left hand. Thus, it is assumed that copying printed letters in longhand indicates that letter images are intact. However, it is possible that correct writing is evoked by other means. Therefore, we must be skeptical about the accuracy of this conclusion in accordance with the above, regarding dictation. Even when the patient only copies written material by drawing from the model, one does not always know whether this is due to alexia or to inability to evoke the writing melody (in which case it is said that the patient "no longer knows how the writing motions are performed".) The latter seems to apply where the patient continues writing after the first letter has been written for him, but even here, the above explanation of arousal by the visual word image cannot be altogether ignored. This is also true when the patient must reflect before writing. Further, letter drawing and free copying occur together. Some patients with adequate self-observation report the "extinction" of the visual and inner-speech components. In such cases we should perhaps discriminate between casual *knowledge* of the form of what is to be written and the incapacity to accomplish the form of movement.

The above contrast in the motor sphere between volition and automatism appears again in the fact that writing monitored by eye is often worse than automatic writing (even with the eyes closed.)

Evaluation of whether the disorder is a *motor form* is helped by accompanying phenomena, characterized as *apraxic*. This form is characteristic of apraxia, as when patients show defects of hand position and of manipulation of the writing implement (which can also be occasionally explained by sensory or sensorimotor disturbances.)

Similarly (i.e. defects in the transfer of the motion melody), passive writing in the air has a supportive effect which prepares the way as practice (although it is possible that this maneuver may also support the emergence of the visual.) More striking are cases where writing again becomes possible on the basis of other similar motions. Moreover, this applies in cases where words are written correctly, but not the constituent letters, or where the name or other signs are written automatically; yet in spite of intact letter comprehension, the letters cannot be combined. In this form of agraphia, writing is generally poor, while in visually determined agraphia, copying and writing from dictation may be better than spontaneous writing. However, even here the relationships are not unambiguous. Patients with adequate self-observation will say that they have the inner word and can spell it, but are incapable of putting it into writing. Occasionally, patients will state that the necessary concentration on the letter form entails difficulties in perceiving the whole picture.

From these various conditions we may draw the theoretical conclusion that the above contrast concerns not so much a rigid "either-or," but only a "both-and" situation.

Indirectly, of course, the absence of any sign of alexia supports the diagnosis. Inability to write with the left hand is not alone proof of a motor genesis, but indicates whether the visual component is preserved, since it is closely bound to learning to write with the left hand. But limited training of the left hand must also be taken into consideration.

The addition of writing, which is difficult in the abstract, accounts for the emergence of paragraphia as a result of fatigue after paraphasia has passed. This also indicates that defects in attentional distribution have a specific effect on the genesis of paragraphia.

The leading influence of the acoustic motor element on the arousal of the motor aspect of writing explains immediately the verbal paragraphic derailments, while similar disturbances developing only in the course of motor writing may explain the more independent literal form.

The close clinical relationship of paragraphia with paraphasia suggests a dependency of the former to the latter. It is attached to the secondary agraphic forms and is dependent on sensory aphasia; accordingly, our entire discussion of paraphasia applies equally to paragraphia.

Two forms are to be distinguished: (1) a form in which writing corresponds to what the patient himself speaks, either aloud or inaudibly; and (2) that in which writing and self-dictation differ. In the former, the normal congruence between speech and writing is preserved, there is "written paraphasia." In the latter, this congruence is disturbed, possibly by the fact that the formulated thought runs ahead of writing. Thus, there is loss of inhibition so that paraphasias derived from slips of the tongue, similar to normal "misreadings," develop only in writing.

The preservation of writing with alexia and/or in the absence of the visual script image, though often difficult to prove, can be explained by the fact that writing, automatized by training, is directly aroused rather than by the script image as in unskilled individuals. There is evidence against the assumption of a "graphic" center in which the "mnemonic images of the motions" of writing are stored and supposedly disturbed in agraphia (Dejerine). Thus, the motor aphasic cannot combine the text with printed letters, because the visual concepts of letters are lacking. This, however, does not affect our interpretation for that center. Nonetheless, it has been demonstrated that in the absence of the corresponding conceptual images, writing may be completely correct (Goldstein and Gelb, 1918). Apart from the role of training, the linguistic type (motor) may play a part. The occasional worse copying in such cases may derive from the greater difficulty of the volitional process compared to the automatized process. Miscopying may be determined by writing what is incorrectly read. Correct copying in the presence of alexia may simply be drawing from the model, its character concealed by the fact that automatic writing is evoked in this way.

In the unskilled writer and individuals who are visually oriented by nature, the disturbance of the script image may be crucial for the occurrence of agraphia.

It is difficult to give a general account of the patient's attitude toward his deficiency since many factors come into play. Each case must be analyzed separately in this respect. The first consideration is, of course, whether alexia is present; such self-deceptions may be caused by the preservation of similar motion structures.

The dependence of writing on speech derives from learning to write and is generally maintained thereafter. This is why every motor-aphasic disorder similarly affects writing, often to the same degree, as well as their parallel course in improvement. This relationship is clarified by cases with the opposite picture, motor aphasia without agraphia from the beginning. Here we may assume that the motor writing structures have become completely emancipated from the speech melodies. This leads to the conclusion that the variable influence of aphemia on writing is due to the degree of this dependence. This is all the more true for deaf-mutes, in whom sign language and writing are even more closely related, as in a published case of agraphia due to motor aphasia (i.e. disorder of gesture language). The exceptional case of severe writing defect in relation to motor aphasia may reflect a marked individual dependence of writing on speech or on other general factors.

From this account of agraphic phenomena associated with aphemia through functional dependence, we must naturally exclude cases where, in accordance with the proximity of the motor centers for speech and writing, the latter is either directly involved in damage of the former or incorporated through proximity effects. Here agraphia is simply a complication of aphemia.

This account of the dependence of writing on speech applies *mutatis mutandis* to the influence of the acoustic components of inner speech, the leading role of which in speech we are already familiar. However, for the discussed relation between paragraphia and paraphasia, only the dependence on disordered speech is plausible. Since word-deafness is not always accompanied by agraphia, which in turn may depend on word-blindness due to the corresponding localization of the lesions, we may say that even the indirect effect of the acoustic component on writing is not very firmly established. Clearly, writing from dictation must be influenced by disorders of the acoustic component, i.e. by varying degrees of speech-deafness.

This is even more pertinent for those disturbances which precede or accompany the transfer of inner speech than for the secondary phenomena. All these disorders of a semiological or morphological nature will also be found in writing, i.e. disorders of sentence meaning as well as of grammatization (motor agrammatism from poverty of speech or separately from poverty of writing, and temporal paragrammatism as a disorder of the feeling for language.) Such differences between speech and writing can be explained from chronological as well as other differences (better writing when the aphemia is still severe.) The striking phenomena of Negersprache on writing from dictation is due to the fact that the patient comprehends the entire sentence, apart from direct copying, and then reproduces it in abbreviated form corresponding to his poverty of speech.

It is self-evident that these semiological disorders, which are secondary effects on writing, can also occur primarily in motor-determined agraphia.

We speak of *amnestic agraphia* when in amnestic aphasia the writing of a word does not take place because it has not occurred to the individual. Goldstein (1910) differentiates an *amnestic form of apraxic agraphia* from this group, in which the volitional impulse does not generate the motion melody due to increased difficulty in arousing the motion scheme. According to that interpretation which rejects the motion scheme, especially in such automatized motions as speaking and writing, we may speak of the impossibility or increased difficulty of their arousal.

Echographia (Pick, 1900; Margulies, 1907; Bernard, 1889) is a rare phenomena characterized by the painstaking and precise copying of all written or printed matter placed before the patient, including nonsensical and foreign language material. The patient makes no effort to respond to written questions or refute insults. This concerns temporal lesions, with agraphia and varying degrees of word-deafness. There may be some disinhibition here as in echolalia, an interpretation consistent with the fact that these phenomena occur together with other forms of echokinesia of a functional or organic-functional character.

There are certain obviously attenuated forms, where the echographia does not give the impression of compulsiveness, but contains a certain element of intention. As supported by the statements of echokinetic patients, there appears to be a mental aftereffect of the original compulsion to continue.

Mirror writing, as in normal (abduction) left-handed writing, is the rule in aphasics and without pathological significance. The occasional interchange between mirror and normal writing, sometimes within the same word, as found in children learning to write, is clearly due to a laxity of the automatic adjustment in the presence of an occasional volitional impulse. Unusual simultaneous training of the left hand during writing with the right and perhaps also other mental factors, e.g. attention directed to the writing, may explain the fact that as in normals left-handed writing is sometimes not in mirror script. A case reported by Bramwell (1897) helps to clarify these contradictions. An agraphic patient wrote his name easily with the left hand in mirror script, but wrote few other words with difficulty in right-handed abduction writing.

In correspondence with the previously mentioned "reverse speech," there are rare cases in which the letters of correctly pronounced words are written in the reverse order (Buchwald, 1878; Wilks, 1879; Erlenmayer, 1879; Peretti, 1882; Ireland, 1882; Dufour, 1903).

To understand the *orthographic disorders,* we must consider the genetic factor and the unequal difficulty in various languages due to differences between phonetic and orthographic writing. Orthography is a late acquisition and is therefore easily impaired. The special nature of the relevant mechanisms is suggested by the isolated occurrence of defective orthography in recovery. This occurs in persons of otherwise high intelligence from inability (often familial) to acquire this function. Its coincidence with congenital reading difficulty indicates the approach of the anatomicophysiological interpretation. It is not known how far the higher functions are involved, say the comprehension of the differentiation of the word meaning, e.g. in German by a circumflex, nor do we know the possible dependence of different phenomena on the typical forms of aphasia.

With regard to the localization of the involved centers, we have discussed the role of the angular gyrus in visually determined writing defects and the foot of F2 for motor disturbances *sensu stricto,* both ordinarily on the left side; the function of the latter center is analogous to that of Broca's area.

Chapter 18

ARITHMETICAL AND NUMERICAL DISORDERS

I<small>N THE BEGINNING</small> we noted the *special position of numbers,* which leads us to devote a few summary remarks on disorders of this important class of signs and their related mental operations.

The *recognition* of numbers may be disordered in the most varied degrees. Two-digit numbers may, for example, be recognized but not those of more than two digits. Patients may name digits better than find them. In the case of numbers of several digits, there is lack of understanding of the significance of position, with fragmentation of the digits in reading. The *writing* of numbers may also be variably disordered with respect to both shape (hooks and loops reversed) and content. Certain numbers (year of birth) may be written but no others. Arabic numerals are recognized and written and not Roman numerals, at least until convalescence. Two-digit numbers are begun with the units digit. *Auditory comprehension* of numbers ordinarily corresponds to that aroused in other ways, rarely worse than word comprehension. Occasionally in recovery, the understanding of numbers preceeds speech. *Arithmetical symbols* are usually not visually recognized at first. They may be confused among themselves or with letters or equated to each other. *Counting* may be preserved without knowledge of the numbers or their meaning as a multiplicity. Similarly, other arithmetical operations may be possible, usually the simpler ones first. Addition alone may be retained with no knowledge of the meaning of other arithmetical operations, or it may also be disordered through ignorance of the direction in which to proceed. As these disorders improve, counting (mentally or on the fingers) comes into play as an aid; the number is understood if it can be counted to (ed. motor series).

In addition, we should mention the misnaming of correctly recognized *coins* and the semantic defect of failure to understand the relative value of coins (Head). (Speech disorders that may simulate arithmetical errors must, of course, be taken into account!) A finding similar to reverse speech (*q.v.*) appears in the occasional reversal of correct digits in multidigit numbers. Sometimes an arithmetical operation (multiplying) with denominated numbers succeeds better than one with pure numbers (evidently assisted by fixation of attention on the object).

The evaluation of these phenomena must begin with the fact that numbers are *ideographic signs* for entities and are therefore firmly established gestalts; both of these features are lacking in letters, since the shape of the letter withdraws in favor of the overall shape of the word. It must also be remembered that the number of digits is considerably smaller than the number of letters. Another difficulty between digits, numbers, and words is that the latter generally have more than one meaning, in contrast to the unambiguity of the former ("monosemic"). These factors produce a priority for digits as compared to both letters and words. Also of importance is the fact that cardinal numbers, as names of primitive concepts (along with the names of body parts), belong to the original vocabulary of speech. Arithmetical signs and their operations behave differently. The symbols have no meaning of their own, as do the subordinate words. Both are late phylogenetic and ontogenetic acquisitions, especially as compared to counting. These factors, rather than a peculiarity of the shape of figures as compared to letters, explain the special position of figures as particularly *resistant* components of aphasic disorders. The special position of the multiplication table (written as well as oral) is explained by its early acquisition and its function as an achievement of serial performance. The significance of this has already been discussed and is compatible with its function as an aid. This situation accounts for other similar disturbances of knowledge acquired later in life, such as the lack of comprehension of the value of position in numbers. The comprehension and reproduction of seen figures and numbers concerns both disorders of the gestalt perception and reproduction and disorders of concepts of direction. (Drawing them from a model occasionally leads to the recognition of compound numbers.) The reversal of two-digit numbers is explained in some languages by the contrast between their linguistic expression and their written form. If the concept which corresponds to the written form is not predominant, they may be written according to the linguistic form. This is seen in the correction of an oral designation which is adapted to the written one. The special position of arithmetical operations appears in the occasional contrast of reading multidigit numbers by means of naming the individual digits, even when there is good comprehension and computation.

Arithmetical disorders due mainly to absence of the number concept concern defects of the intellectual functions and frequently occur with temporo-occipital lesions, less often with frontal lesion. Thus, they primarily involve visual imagery and gestalt perception. In frontal lesions, defects of counting are prominent. An important role is played by memory disorders (forgetting the nature of the problem) and attentional distribution. Also important are distractability, poor concentration, and forgetfulness of component operations, component results, and the major task (memory is variable in different functional areas, and thus there is the possibility of compensatory function.)

We still lack a detailed psychological analysis of the different arithmetical operations which could provide a framework for their understanding. Presumably, more detailed pathological studies will contribute to such an analysis. The arithmetical operations are associated with certain relationships; lack of comprehension of the operations, in the form of undeveloped awareness of their relationships, is reminiscent of analogous disorders of sensory (impressive) agrammatism, in which terms indicating relationships are commonly not understood. Similarly, otherwise automatized arithmetical operations are disturbed by the necessity of resorting to the linguistic component, which is itself disordered. Mental arithmetic succeeds better than written. Minor calculations may be done automatically, without need of the patient's confidence. Counting may be correct in spite of paraphasic slips of the tongue. In accordance with our knowledge of mental arithmeticians, differences in mental types are decisive (mental images, visual or other schemata) as well as individual methods (simultaneous speech, the aid of mental images.)

From these observations, there appears to be no need to assume special centers for figures and numbers, as within the visual-psychic centers already present; such centers in Wernicke's or Broca's region appear untenable. We are dealing here with basically similar functions. For now there can be no question of differentiation of the involved functional territories in the various arithmetical operations. The fact of greater importance of the left hemisphere, even for sensory functions, agrees with the observation that disorders in computation appear to be more frequent with lesions of the left side, especially of the angular gyrus region.

Chapter 19

CLINICAL FORMS

IN ORDER TO RELATE our discussion thus far with a schematically oriented clinical point of view, if only as to nomenclature, we must append a brief discussion of the clinical forms on the basis of Wernicke's diagram (Fig. 2).

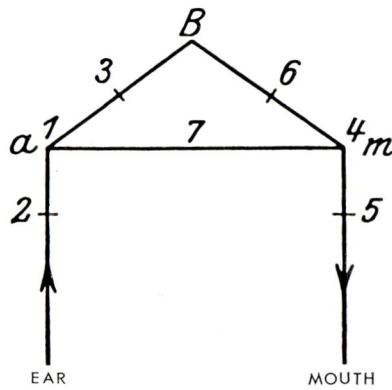

Figure 2. Wernicke's diagram of aphasia: B = Concept field, the entire cortex except for the speech zone. 1. Cortical sensory aphasia. 2. Subcortical sensory aphasia. 3. Transcortical sensory aphasia. 4. Cortical motor aphasia. 5. Subcortical motor aphasia. 6. Transcortical motor aphasia. 7. Conduction aphasia.

These may be divided into the categories of *motor (frontal)* and *sensory (temporal) aphasia,* with the qualifications that in the latter actual sensory symptoms may be absent in a particular stage.

The complete type of the former is *Broca's (cortical motor) aphasia, aphemia,* with its consequences for reading and writing. It corresponds to a lesion of the pars opercularis of F3, while it is uncertain whether there need be involvement of adjacent parts, in particular the pars triangularis. The proximity of this region to the pars opercularis of Ca, the seat of the motor centers, explains the complication of dysarthric disorders (functionally or anatomically determined.) The presumed regularity of secondary aftereffects has been explained on the basis of destruction of "motor memory images" in the cortical center. Accordingly, *pure aphemia,* which does not show such aftereffects, has been attributed to a *subcortical* localization. Both the theoretical basis of this account and its postulated pathoanatomical implications have been demonstrated to be unconvincing. Rather, the clinical differences depend on the severity and extent of the primary lesion, its diaschitic effects, and on the autonomization of the secondary speech elements, as evidenced chiefly by the transition from the one form to the others.

This is also true for the third form, *transcortical motor aphasia* (transcortical in the sense that the lesion is supposed to be situated beyond the cortical center.) Characteristically and in accordance with the assumed discontinuity between the concept (psychic) center and the motor speech center, spontaneous speech is said to be severely impaired with constant echolalia. But this combination occurs in both typical Broca's aphasia and as a stage in its recovery.

Analogus relationships occur in the sensory forms; as in typical *Wernicke's (cortical sensory) aphasia, word-deafness,* with its consequence of paraphasia and its secondary effects in reading and writing. This condition involves that part of the first temporal convolution situated anterior to Heschl's convolution (though it is questionable how far toward the center of the first convolution), just rostral to which in that convolution is located the musical acoustic center. The proximity of the temporal transverse convolutions, Heschl's convolutions, as the actual acoustic center accounts for the simulation of analogous symptoms due to partial cortical deafness. This is also true of labyrinthine deafness. *"Pure" word-deafness, subcortical sensory aphasia,* in which the absence of secondary effects on reading and writing were also explained on the subcortical localization (No. 2), has been found to be a fabrication not correlated with observation (even in symmetrical cortical lesions located in both temporal lobes; the recovery form is typical cortical sensory aphasia.)

This also applies to *transcortical sensory aphasia,* which according to the diagram was supposed to differ from the cortical form in the different behavior with respect to echoing. This has also been found to be determined by partial compensation or improvement of the cortical form with a similar localization.

The last schematic construction was *conduction aphasia* abandoned later by Wernicke himself (No. 7). The principal feature was assumed to be disordered conductance between the acoustic and motor parts of the speech processes, themselves intact, due to lesion of the pathway situated in the island of Reil. This concerns predominantly the attenuated forms of cortical sensory aphasia; the question of involvement of Broca's area is undecided. Besides Broca's and Wernicke's aphasia, which thus appear to be the only established forms, this applies also to *total* (ed. global) *aphasia,* due to lesion of both territories (temporary obscuration of the temporal speech disorder by the more severe frontal one, aphemia, early return of speech-deafness.) The forms of *pure alexia* and *agraphia* also appear to be clinically established; in regard to these, the reader is referred to our previous discussion concerning localization in the description of symptomatology.

Amnestic aphasia is firmly established as an additional form, although not expained by the old scheme, or only by an artificial interpretation. For this entity and its localization, the reader again is referred to the previous discussion. It frequently occurs as an accompaniment of other lesions, but this is not inconsistent with the localization to which clinico-anatomical and psychological considerations have lead, since we account for it by slight involvement of the temporal lobe and by the relatively difficult function of word-finding.

Our anatomical description regarding these clinical forms must be quite general. There is little agreement on even the least particular as it is impossible to bring the microscopic findings into harmony with the nature and extent of the disorders.

Chapter 20

GESTURE LANGUAGE

W<small>E HAVE CHARACTERIZED</small> speech as a highly developed system of expression developed phylo and ontogenetically from the cry, supported by pantomime and gesture which are indispensable to it in certain aspects. Thus, it may be that at a certain stage in development, extending chronologically farther back than speech, there may also be *pathology* of this means of expression. In this connection it must be remembered that even ontogenetically both precede the stage of verbalization. *Pantomime* is largely excluded here as a mainly involuntary expression of feelings and bound to subcortical mechanisms. Only that aspect of pantomime which as a more or less voluntary innervation contributes to the expression of meaningful gestures, such as nodding the head in affirmation, shaking the head in negation, is to be considered separately here. However, it would be a mistake to underestimate these forms of expression as a part of speech. We have discussed differences in the pantomime of aphasics and noted that many aphasics cannot accomplish even the pantomime of affirmation and negation, or they may confuse the two, thereby exhibiting a semantic functional disturbance similar to their confusion of the linguistically produced "yes" and "no." The occasional disorders of voluntary innervation of the facial musculature observed with this phenomenon provide a transition to the area of apraxia, the explanation of which begins historically with these very phenomena. The position of pantomime and gesture within the framework of aphasia is clarified by the fact that in cases of severe aphemia both are commonly exaggerated as a compensation. The second system of means of expression, developed into a volitional system and phylogenetically preceding actual speech, is *sign* or *gesture language,* the *language of primitives* and of *deafmutes who have not been taught to speak*. In ethnic differentiation, however, this forms a more or less learned accompaniment of spoken language. (Loss of gesture sometimes occurs with total aphasia and also with motor aphasia.) It is not known why in recovery a poverty of the entire sign language appears with the occurrence of unintelligible gestures. The preservation of *emotional pantomime* and *gesture* in such cases is understandable. Rarely observed is the *lack of understanding of gestures*. An account of the details of sign languages, certainly a mine of information for pathological semiology, would be out of place here, since at the present time we can deduce little from it because of the extremely scanty pathology. It is evident that these are not merely conventionally developed utterances from the close similarity between the gestures of savages and deaf-mutes, such as enables them to communicate directly with each other. This primitivity of language accounts for the rarity of such disorders in persons of normal intelligence (Ribot's rule). The psychological analogy with spoken language appears established, since the linguistic sign corresponds originally not to the single word, but to the whole sentence. It is clear that the study of the language of deaf-mutes with school education can greatly aid our understanding of the many aspects of expressive motor agrammatism and similar disorders of speech development (syntax of sign language) and sensory agrammatism (comprehension of speech without auxiliary words.) Even the deaf-mute or blind deaf-mute untrained in speech involuntarily accompanies his formulated thought with often visible finger movements. From these, both spontaneously and with instruction, a practical system of signs for communication develops, which are expressed in movements of the upper extremities and supported as in normals by pantomime. Here again, childhood imitation plays a part, as shown by observations of the children of deaf-mutes.

Rarely, one sees deaf-mutes untrained in speech (Grasset, Burr) who, as might be expected, have lost their usual sign language following lesion of the left hemisphere (no autopsy findings are available). Despite intact motility of the fingers, such patients may lose only the sign language of the right hand. The impressive part of speech may be similarly disturbed. One patient was unable to read letters of the deaf-mute alphabet with the right hand though able to do so with the left. It may be that in such cases the expressive disorder is due (by analogy with motor aphasia and agraphia) to a lesion anterior to the hand center. The function of this area can be explained according to the above analogy, with the qualification that we are dealing here not with similar processes but with simpler processes, so that this center may coincide spatially with that in the foot of F2. For the impressive disorder, a portion of the visuopsychic area (parieto-occipital region) may be involved. This may also be true for the above-mentioned lack of understanding of gestures occurring with aphasia.

Chapter 21

AMUSIA

SPEECH AND SINGING have a common phylogenetic development (first emotional sounds, only later music) and largely employ the same peripheral executive and perceptual organs. Thus, they differ in the manner of modifications of the same function. Their boundary has been shown to be fluid, since speech, unlike music which is entirely autonomous, cannot dispense with musical elements as an important functional supplement. These aid in the expression of emotions, and speech suffers in various ways, as we have seen, from their disorder. We grasp the full significance of the musical components of speech, especially for the semiological aspect of aphasia theory, when we consider that in certain languages (e.g. Chinese) the meaning of homonymous words differs with different intonation. This makes it appear a priori probable that the two cerebral mechanisms, though not identical, are situated in close topological relationship. This is confirmed by the frequent occurrence of these disorders both together and separately. When the musical processes are affected alone, the disorders are grouped together as amusia. The frequent concurrence of the two series, in addition to the above, explains why the same categories of aphasia and the schemas to which they lead are also found within the framework of amusia. They find their bases in *disorders of musical production (vocal* and *instrumental), of musical comprehension, of the ability to read and write musical notation (note alexia* and *note agraphia.)* These disorders obviously run parallel to the aphasias and individually or jointly affect the category of tones (pitch, volume, timbre), melody, rhythm, and the expression of feeling; in addition, there may be differences between expressive and impressive disorders (e.g. retention of ability to sing with loss of the ability to read music, analogous to isolated alexia.) A detailed account, therefore, is unnecessary in the framework of this monograph, since we know even less about the processes underlying these disorders and their anatomical basis than about the corresponding aphasic disorders. Moreover, they are less frequently isolated than in combination with aphasia, and that which is most pertinent to these combinations has already been discussed. In addition, the amusias show no lack of parallels to the congenital defects which were encountered in aphasia. Certainly, we cannot overestimate the importance of an investigation of amusia, especially as the methods available for such an investigation are far superior to those of aphasia theory in precision and clarity. However, we must attend to the fact that some of these phenomena (tempo, rhythm, modulation) involve functions whose participation (basal ganglia, cerebellum) has hardly been considered heretofore (Gutzman, Isserlin). This is suggested by the simultaneous occurrence of disorders of musical tempo and dancing (Edgren, 1903). The conclusion regarding the involved cerebral areas has been confirmed by anatomical observations. The center corresponding to expressive vocal disorders is probably situated in F3, anterior to Broca's area and that corresponding to instrumental disorders in F2 bilaterally. The center for the impressive side of music appears to be anterior to Wernicke's area in T1, while disorders of music reading and writing probably coincide with lesions in the inferior parietal lobule. With regard to certain of these disorders (tone deafness), the leading role of the left hemisphere has again been demonstrated. The localization of the capacity for musical expression appears to be established in the right hemisphere, from a few cases with brain lesions of the right side. These cases suggest that both hemispheres are involved in singing, but that a lesion of either one impairs the function. As in speech development in the child, the musical elements of speech are among the earliest to be acquired and the most automatized. This is also true of singing, which is more permanently bound to both hemispheres than is speech. The fact that aphemia and motor amusia do not necessarily coincide is not evidence of a separation of the two centers. Rather, it is to be explained by a functional differentiation of a common center. The bilateral arrangement appears to be in inverse proportion to the level of development. In instrumental amusia, the technique is of course decisive and in both hemispheres concerns the foot of F2 and probably also F3.

In this regard, certain factors concerned in the so-called musical components of speech should be mentioned. Although these are part of phonology, they also represent a frequent component of aphasic disorders, insofar as modulated speech, i.e. ordinary speech, has a musical accompaniment. Both in expressive and impressive speech these components are extraordinarily resistant as compared to others. This is due to their (phylo and ontogenetic) chronological priority and their consequent greater automatization. This is shown by the rare and delayed loss of the emotional speech. Also, in certain of these factors (tempo, rhythm, intonation), evidently because of their emotional basis, different anatomical foundations are involved (basal ganglia, cerebellum, connections with the temporal lobe through Türck's bundle.) Also of importance, especially with regard to localization, is in what part of the speech process the various musical components come into play. For the emotionally determined components, the stage of mental formulation certainly is involved from which the whole intonational pattern develops. The most important of these aspects were discussed with the aphasic disorders. We should also mention the importance of intonation for correct comprehension, even of reading where some guidance is provided by the normal case. Not only the individual type but also ethnic differences will be important, depending on the singing quality of the language or dialect.

The close relationships found between the two sets of phenomena and their basic similarity suggests (disregarding the fact that singing requires the motility of other organs besides those of speech), that the relationships are not sharply differentiated functional categories but overlapping neuronal pools interconnected in different ways for different activities. However, even within the musical centers, no sharp topographical boundaries can be drawn, nor can we, for example, assume one special center for notes and another for clefs. It is clear that the same explanation also holds for any separation of special instrumental musical centers from those of music in general. The assumption of a varying assemblage of more or less automatized motion combinations is sufficient.

This is also true for the relationships between music-deafness, noise-deafness, and word-deafness, different types of disorders of a largely unitary region.

Chapter 22

APHASIA AND INTELLIGENCE

THE CLOSE RELATIONSHIPS between the mental and the physical which have been discussed and differentiated in this work suggest the propriety of touching briefly on the equally important question of the intelligence of aphasics, thereby shedding some light on a separate field of research in psychophysical relationships.

There are special difficulties in the concept of the nonidentity of thought and speech, even for a rough appraisal of the problem. This is because the question of whether there is a *direct connection* or merely a *complication,* the evaluation of anatomicophysiological secondary effects, can rarely be precisely solved, even in stationary cases. However, apart even from this, the problem is further obscured by our inability to demarcate once and for all between verbal and nonlinguistic thought. This question divides into two parts, practical or scientific. If we define intelligence as the capacity to adapt to the social requirements, we can generally observe a *difference between patients with frontal and temporal aphasias*. In the former, if no complication is present, the mental capacity generally appears unimpaired, but there is damage to the mechanism by which the various sides of mental activity serving for verbalization are brought into play. Processes which occur in the temporal lobe are closer in regard to both expressive and impressive speech to those which run parallel to the mental *sensu stricto* (e.g. think of the great difficulty experienced by the speech-deaf patient in grasping the *situation* developing between him and the speaker, and of the disturbing effect of the lack of this development on his intellectual comprehension of the content expressed in speech.) Accordingly, barring recovery, it is particularly the sensory forms that are accompanied by severe intellectual disorder. It is not accidental nor merely due to the apparent (linguistic) confusion that an extraordinarily large number of such cases still go to psychiatric clinics. However, anatomically proven cases are known, with recovery, of persons of high intellectual standing, where even the higher demands of everyday life could be satisfied. Recently, a case of total aphasia was reported (Vernet and Merland, 1922) in which the dementia is only apparent. A useful criterion concerns the above-mentioned facts regarding the varying attitude of the patient towards his deficiency, inasmuch as this permits a conclusion, according to the degree of the deficiency, as to the level of critical perception of which the total personality is capable. This criterion must be used with caution, however, since an intact attitude may be found in combination with a decline from a former high intellectual position.

Similarly, we interpret as *secondary* (narrowed span of awareness, defects of attentional distribution) though often also as primary those disorders which affect the combination of words into a sentence, the correct sequence in reproduction, and retention of the "thread" and its goal necessary for that purpose. In *disorders of inner speech* it is particularly *abstract, conceptual thought* which suffers. Thus, primarily those activities are affected whose object, for want of other physical content, takes hold of the words that denote it. This is in accord with the effect of amnestic aphasia (Lotmar, Ach). Conversely, Ach (1921) showed that some of his patients had not lost the *formation* of concepts, that this is independent of the brain defect underlying the speech disorder. One polyglot with a strong visual imagination (Charcot; Pick, 1923) showed, following lesion in the visuopsychic area, an impairment (subjective) of thinking in a later-learned language.

Recently, Fischer described *personality changes* (a peculiar submissiveness and politeness) in women with transcortical sensory aphasia; however, in such changes the question of a *complication* cannot be answered at the present time.

This question appears still more difficult when considered from the scientific point of view. Our knowledge of the semiological aspect of aphasia is too scanty to permit a sharp demarcation of the intellectual and indicates the need for more precise study of this side of the problem (Head).

The *repercussions of aphasic disorders,* which are to be interpreted as *secondary,* are better known but can only be clarified by examples. They are mainly explained by the fact that speech symbols represent an important *aid to thought* in the more complex abstract operations. We cannot detail here the extent to which disorders of intellectual tools influence intelligence itself, but can only offer a few indications. In general we may say that the influence of linguistic patterns on thought development (Selz, 1922) in normals suggests an analogous situation in pathological cases. Thus, wherever the assistance of the disordered linguistic accompaniments is necessary or utilized, its deficiency has a more or less damaging effect (Goldstein, Lotmar, Head). On the other hand, the Countess von Kuenburg was able to show that even in severe cases of motor or sensory aphasia, the comprehension of relationships is intact and only the reproduction appears disordered.

Isserlin (1931) has shown that in the acquisition of new linguistic memory, the speech motor disorder, which may be barely noticed, still has a disturbing effect ("aphasic defect of memory").

In this regard, it should also be mentioned that in the course of the stage-by-stage linguistic formulation of thought, discussed earlier, the part already formulated influences the course of the thought, so that the disturbance may produce the appearance of a mental deficiency more apparent than real.

Moreover, the theory of Marie (according to which intellectual disorders of a special nature underly aphasic phenomena) has, except for his school, been quite generally rejected (Dejerine, 1906; Lotmar and Montet, 1906; Liepmann, 1909; Chatelin, 1918; Foix, 1921).

Chapter 23

CONCLUDING REMARKS

IN THE FOREGOING, an attempt has been made to collate all that can presumably contribute to a dynamic conception of the individual phenomena and processes. Insofar as the purpose of the Handbook permits, different aspects have been presented on which the relationships between the above are based as they appear in the various clinical forms.

Even more than the clinical picture, methods of treatment are beyond the scope of this Handbook. However, since most treatment has the purpose of retraining the functions that remain intact or those in recovery, our functional point of view may provide a proper basis for those methods. The presentation, to be sure, has highlighted the gaps and obscurities almost more than the extent of our knowledge. Only after these gaps have been more accurately appraised, and where possible filled in through correct methodology, and with the support of more advanced anatomicophysiological observations, shall be able to proceed to the construction, premature at this time, of a system of the purely endogenous aphasic disorders determined by impairment of the psychic speech apparatus as a part of a psychophysiology of the brain.

BIBLIOGRAPHY*

1. Ach, N.: *Über die Begriffsbildung.* Buchner, Hamburg, 1921, 3, 13.*
2. Alt, F.: *Melodientaubheit und musikalisches Falschhören.* Wien, 1906, 21.*
3. Asayama, T.: Über die Aphasie bei Japanern. *Dtsch. Arch. klin. Med., 113*:523-529, 1914.
4. Balassa, L.: Zur Psychologie der Seelentaubheit. *Dtsch. Z. Nervenheilk., 77*:153, 1923, 15, 21.*
5. Ballet, G.: *Die innerliche Sprache und die verschiedenen Formen der Aphasie.* transl. P. Bongers., Deuticke, Leipzig, 1890, 7.*
6. Barat, L. and Chaslin: Le langage, in *Traite de Psychologie, Dumas* (Ed.) *1*:733, 1923, 1.*
7. Benary, W.: Studien zur Untersuchung der Intelligenz bei einem Fall von Seelenblindheit. *Psychol Forsch., 2*:209-297, 1922, 18, 22.*
8. Bergson, H.: *Matière et mémoire.* Paris, 1896.
9. Bernard, O.: *De l'aphasie et ses diverses formes.* Lecrosnier et Babe, Paris, 1889.
10. Bernheim, F.: *L'aphasie motrice.* Paris, 1900, 4.*
11. Bezold, F.: Demonstration einer kontinuierlichen Tonreihe zum Nachweis von Gehördefekten, etc. *Ztschr. Psychol., 13*:161-174, 1897, 15.*
12. Bianchi, L.: *La meccanica del cervello e la funzione dei lobi frontale.* Bocca, Torino, 1920, 22.*
13. Bianchi, L.: Le syndrome parietale. *Acta Otolaryngol., 8*:353-363, 1925, 22.*
14. Bonhoeffer, K.: Zur Kenntnis der Rückbildung motorischer Aphasien. *Mitt. aus den Grenzgeb. Med. der Chir., 10*:203, 1902, 14.*
15. Bonhoeffer, K.: Zur Klinik und Lokalisation des Agrammatismus und der Rechts-Links-Desorientierung. *Mschr. Psychiat. u. Neurol., 54*:11-42, 1923, 14.*
16. Bonvicini, G.: Über bilaterale Apraxie der Gesichts-und Sprachmuskulatur. *Jahrb.f.Psychiat.u.Neurol., 36*:563-630, 1914, 20.*
17. Book: *The psychology of will,* 1908.
18. Bouman, L. and Grünbaum, A.: Experimentell-psychologische Untersuchungen zur Aphasie und Paraphasie.*Ztschr.f.d.Ges.Neur.U.Psychiat., 96*:481-538, 1925, 22.*
19. Bramwell, B.: Lectures on aphasia. *Edinb.Med.J., 44*:1, 1897.
20. Brissaud, E.: *Rev.neurol.,* 101, 1904.
21. Broadbent, W.: A case of peculiar affection of speech with commentary. *Brain, 1*:484-503, 1878, 14.*
22. Broca, P.: Remarques sur le siège de la faculté de langage articulé, suivies

---

* Those references not mentioned in the text pertain, in the original, to the general subject of each chapter. This is indicated by an asterisk following these entries.

d'une observation d'aphémie (perte de la parole). *Bull.Soc.Anat., 36*: 330-357, 1861a, 4.*
23. Broca, P.: Nouvelle observation d'aphémie produite une lésion de la moitié postérieure des deuxième et troisième circonvolutions frontales. *Bull.Soc.Anat., 36*:398-407, 1861b, 4.*
24. Broca, P.: Mémoire sur le cerveau de l'homme et des primates. In Siège *de la faculté de langage articulé*, pp. 1-62, 1888, 4.*
25. Buchwald: Spiegelschrift bei Hirnkranken. *Berl.klin.Wschr.*, 6, 1878.
26. Bühler, C.: Über Gedankenenstehung. *Ztschr. Psychol., 80*:129, 1918, 6.*
27. Bühler, C.: Über die Prozesse der Satzbildung. *Ztschr. Psychol., 81*:181, 1919, 6.*
28. Bühler, K.: Über Gedanken. *Arch. f. Psychol., 9*:297-365, 1907, 6.*
29. Bühler, K.: Über Gedankenzusammenhange. *Arch. f. Physiol., 12*:1-23, 1908, 5.*
30. Bühler, K.: Über das Sprachverständnis vom Standpunkt der Normalpsychologie. *Berichte über III Kongr. f. exper. Psychol.* Barth, Munich, 1909, 5.*
31. Bühler, K.: *Forschr. Psychol., 3*:294, 1923.
32. Bühler, K.: *Die geistige Entwicklung des Kindes.* Fischer, Jena, 1930, 3.*
33. Chatelin: *Les blessures du cerveau.* Paris, 1918.
34. Collier, W.: Über experimentelle Hypertrophie von Nervenzellen. *J. Med. Res.Boston.*, 439, 1920/21.
35. Davidenkoff, S.: *Rev. neurol.* 12, 1914, 22.*
36. Dejerine, J.: *Sémiologie des affections du système nerveux.* Masson, Paris, 1914, 4, 16.*
37. Dejerine, J.: L'aphasie sensorielle et l'aphasie motrice. *Presse méd., 14*:437-439, 453-457, 1906, 4.*
38. Delbruck, A.: Begriffsgruppen. *Jena Z. Naturwiss., 20*:94, 1887.
39. Dufour, A.: Un cas d'ecriture en miroir. *Rev.med.Suisse rom., 23*:618, 1903.
40. Dupre and Nathan, M.: *Le langage musical.* Lisbon, 1906, 21.*
41. Dyminski: *Über Störungen im Hersagen gelaufiger Reihen bei einem Aphasischen.* Diss. Würzburg, 1908, 12.*
42. Edgren, J.: Amusie (musikalische Aphasie). *Dtsch.Z.Nervenheilk., 6*:1-64, 1895.
43. Egger, V.: *La parole interieure.* Baill, Paris, 1888, 7.*
44. Eliasberg, W.: Die Schwierigkeiten intellektueller Vorgänge und ihre Beziehungen zur Intelligenzpruefung. *Schweiz.Arch.f.Psychiat.u.Neurol., 12*:136-143, 1923.
45. Erdmann, B.: Die psychologischen Grundlagen der Beziehungen zwischen Sprechen und Denken. *Arch.f.system.Philos., 2*:355, 1896; *3*:31, 1897; *7*:147, 1901, 6.*
46. Erdmann, B. and Dodge, R.: *Psychologische Untersuchungen über das Lesen.* Niemeyer, Halle, 1898, 16.*

47. Erlenmeyer: *Die Schriftrundzüge, ihre Psychologie und Pathologie.* Stuttgart, 1879.
48. Feuchtwanger, E.: *Amusie. Studien zur pathologischen Psychologie der akustischen Wahrnehmung und Vorstellung und ihrer Strukturgebiete besonders in Musik und Sprache.* Springer, Berlin, 1930, 21.*
49. Fildes, L.: A psychological inquiry into the nature of the condition known as congenital word-blindness. *Brain, 44*:286-307, 1921.
50. Finkelnburg, F.: Niederrheinische Gesellschaft; Sitzung vom 21 Marz 1870, Bonn. *Berl.klin.Wschr., 7*:449-450, 460-462, 1870, 20.*
51. Fischer, S.: Über das Entstehen und Verstehen von Namen, etc. *Arch.f. Psychol., 42*:335-368; *43*:32-63, 1922, 5, 15.*
52. Fischer, S.: Veranderung psychischer Funktionen bei transcorticaler sensorischer Aphasie. *Berlin.klin.Wschr., 2*:870, 1923, 22.*
53. Förster, E.: Über Amusie. *Allg.Z.Psychiat., 71*:529, 1914, 21.*
54. Förster, E.: Ein Fall von motorischer Amusie. *Neur.Zbl., 37*:437, 1918, 21.*
55. Förster, R.: Agrammatismus, etc. *Mschr. f.Psychiat.u.Neurol., 56*:1, 1918, 14.*
56. Freund, C.: Über optische Aphasie und Seelenblindheit. *Arch.Psychiat. Nervenkr., 20*:276-297, 371-416, 1889, 13.*
57. Freund, C.: *Labrynthtaubheit und Sprachtaubheit.* 1895, 15.*
58. Freund, C.: Labyrnthtaubheit und Grundlagen der Worttaubheit. *Dtsch. Z.Nervenheilk., 35*:25, 1908.
59. Froeschels, E.: Kindersprache und Aphasie. *Abh. aus der Neurol.Psychiat. Psychol., V*:3, 1918, 1, 6.*
60. Froment, J.: Des diverses conceptions de l'aphasie. *J.Méd.Lyon*, 1921, 1.*
61. Froment, J. and Monod: L'épreuve de Proust-Lichtheim-Dejerine. *Rev. méd., 33*:280, 1913, 9.*
62. Gehuchten, P. van and Van Gorp: *Bull.Acad.Med.Belg.*, Marz 1914, 19.*
63. Gelb, A. and Goldstein, K.: Über Farbennamenamnesie. *Forsch.Psychol., 6*:127-186, 1924, 13.*
64. Giannulli, F.: *Riv. di Sper. Freniatr., 40*:145, 1914.
65. Goldscheider, A. and Müller, R.: Zur Physiologie und Pathologie des Lesens. *Ztschr.klin.Med., 23*:131-167, 1893, 16.*
66. Goldstein, K.: Zur Frage der amnestischen Aphasie. *Archiv.f.Psychiat.u. Neurol., 41*:911, 1906, 13.*
67. Goldstein, K.: Über Aphasie. *Beiheft d.mediz.Klinik., 6*:1-32, 1910, 1.*
68. Goldstein, K.: Über eine amnestische Form der apraktischen Agraphie. *Neur.Zbl., 29*:252, 1910.
69. Goldstein, K.: Über die amnestischen und zentrale Aphasie (Leitungsaphasie). *Archiv,f.Psychiat.u.Neurol., 48*:314-343, 1911, 13.*
70. Goldstein, K.: Die zentrale Aphasie. *Neurol.Zbl., 12*:739-751, 1912, 7.*
71. Goldstein, K.: Die Topik der Grosshirnrinde in ihrer klinischen Bedeutung. *Dtsch.Z.Nervenheilk., 77*:12, 1912, 8, 16.*
72. Goldstein, K.: Über die Störungen der Grammatik bei Hirnkrankheiten. *Mschr.f.Psychiat.u.Neur., 34*:540-568, 1913, 14.*

73. Goldstein, K.: *Die transcorticalen Aphasien.* G. Fischer, Jena, 1915, 8, 10, 12, 15.*
74. Goldstein, K.: Das Wesen der amnestischen Aphasie. *Schweiz.Arch.f.Neur. u.Psychiat., 15*:163-175, 1924, 13.*
75. Goldstein, K.: Über Aphasie. *Schweiz.Archiv.f.Neur.u.Psychiat., 19*:3-38, 1926, 1.*
76. Goldstein, K.: Die Lokalisation in der Grosshirnrinde. *Handb.norm. u.path. Physiol., 10*:600-842, 1927.
77. Goldstein, K. and Gelb, A.: Psychologische Analysen hirnpathologischer Falle I. *Ztschr.f.d.ges.Neur.u.Psychiat., 41*:1-142, 1918, 16.*
78. Grashey: Über Aphasie und ihre Beziehungen zur Wahrnehmung. *Arch.f. Psychiat.u.Nervenkr., 16*:654-688, 1885.
79. Grasset, H.: Aphasie de la main droite chez un sourd-muet. *Progres. méd., 4*:281, 1896, 20.*
80. Gross, O.: Biologie des Sprachapparates. *Ztschr.Neurol.u.Psychiat., 61*:795, 1904, 20.*
81. Gutzman, H.: Über Gewohnung und Gewohnheit. *Fortschr.Psychol., 2*:137, 1913.
82. Gutzmann, H.: *Psychologie der Sprache.* Handb.d.vergleich.Psychol., Kafka, 1922, 20.*
83. Head, H.: Aphasia and kindred disorders of speech. *Brain, 43*:87-165, 1920, 1.*
84. Head, H.: On release. *Proc.R.Soc.Lond., 92*:184, 1921, 9.*
85. Head, H.: Speech and speech localization. *Brain, 46*:355-528, 1923.
86. Head, H.: *Aphasia and Kindred Disorders of Speech.* Macmillan, New York, 1926, 1, 6, 22.*
87. Heilbronner, K.: Studien über eine eklamptische Psychose. *Mschr.f. Psychiat.u.Neur., 17*:277, 367, 425, 1905, 11.*
88. Heilbronner, K.: Über Haftenbleiben und Stereotypie. *Mschr.f.Psychiat. u.Neurol., 18*:293-371, 1905, 11.*
89. Heilbronner, K.: Zur Frage der motorischen Asymbolie. *Ztschr.Psychol., 39*:168, 1905, 12.*
90. Heilbronner, K.: Über Agrammatismus und die Störungen der inneren Sprache. *Archiv.f.Psychiat., 41*:653, 1906, 14.*
91. Heilbronner, K.: Die aphasischen, apraktischen und agnostischen Störungen. In Lewandowsky (Ed.): *Handb.d.Neurol., 1*:982-1093, 1910, 12.*
92. Henschen, S.: Über die Hörsphäre. *J.f.Psychol.u.Neur., 22*:319-474, 1917, 15.*
93. Henschen, S.: Über Sprach-, Musik, und Rechenmechanismen und ihre Lokalisation im Grosshirn. *Zschr.f.d.ges.Neur.u.Psychiat., 52*:273-298, 1919, 18.*
94. Henschen, S.: *Klinische und anatomische Beiträge zur Pathologie des Gehirns,* Vols. 5-7. Nordiska, Stockholm, 1920-1922, 1, 5, 8, 12, 13, 15, 16, 18, 21.*

95. Herrmann, G.: Zur Lehre von der motorischen Amusie. *Ztschr.f.d.ges. Neur.u.Psychiat., 93*:95, 1924, 21.*
96. Herrmann, G.: Beiträge zur Lehre von den Störungen des Rechnens bei Herderkrankungen des Okzipitallappens (Akalkulie Henschen). *Mschr. f.Psychiat. u.Neur., 70*:193-278, 1928, 18.*
97. Herrmann, G. and Pötzl, O.: *Über die Agraphie und ihre lokaldiagnostischen Beziehungen.* S. Karger, Berlin, 1926, 17.*
98. Hinshelwood, J.: *Letter-, word- and mind-blindness.* Lewis, London, 1900.
99. Ingenieros: *Les aphasias musicales. Icon de la Salpetriere, 19*:362, 1906, 21.*
100. Ireland: On mirror-writing and its relation to left-handedness and cerebral disease *Brain, 4*:361, 1882.
101. Isserlin, M.: Psychologisch-phonetische Untersuchungen. I. *Ztschr.f.allgem.Psychiat., 75*:1, 1919, 21.*
102. Isserlin, M.: Über Agrammatismus. *Ztschr.f.d.ges.Neur.u.Psychiat., 75*:332-410, 1922, 14.*
103. Isserlin, M.: Über Störungen des Gedachtnisses bei Hirngeschadigten. *Ztschr.f.d.ges.Neur.u.Psychiat., 85*:84-97, 1923.
104. Isserlin, M.: *Ztschr. Neur., 94*:437, 1925.
105. Isserlin, M.: Die pathologische Physiologie der Sprache. *Ergeb.d.Physiol., 29*:129-249, 1929, 1.*
106. Jackson, H.: *Selected Writings of.,* J. Taylor (Ed.), 2 vol., Hodder and Stoughton, London, 1932, 10.*
107. Jossman, P.: Die Beziehungen der motorischen Amusie zu den apraktischen Störungen, *Mschr.f.Psychiat.u.Neur., 63*:239, 1927, 21.*
108. Kehrer, F.: Beiträge zur Aphasielehre mit besonderer Berücksichtigung der amnestischen Aphasie. *Archiv.f.Psychiat., 52*:103, 1913, 10, 13.*
109. Kleist, K.: Über Leitungsaphasie. *Mschr.f.Psychiat.u.Neur., 17*:503, 1905, 14.*
110. Kleist, K.: Über Leitungsaphasie und grammatische Störungen. *Mschr.f. Psychiat.u.Neur., 40*:118-121, 1916, 14.*
111. Kleist, K.: Gehirnverletzungen, ihre Bedeutung fur die Lokalisation der Hirnfunktionen. *Ztschr.f.d.ges.Neur.u.Psychiat., 16*:336, 1918, 18.*
112. Kleist, K.: Gehirnpathologische und lokalisatorische Ergebnisse. 3. Mitteilung: Über sensorische Aphasien. *J.f.Psychol.u.Neur., 37*:146-156, 1928, 15, 21.*
113. Kleist, K.: Gehirnpathologische und lokalisatorische Ergebnisse über Hörstörungen. Gerauschtaubheiten und Amusien. *Mschr.f.Psychiat.u. Neur., 68*:853-860, 1928, 15, 21.*
114. Klemm, O.: Wahrnemungsanalyse: in Abderhaldens *Handb.d.physiol. Arbeitsmeth., 6*:1, 1921.
115. Knoblauch, A.: Über Störungen der musikalischen Leistungsfähigkeit infolge von Gehirnläsionen. *Dtsch.Arch.klin.Med., 43*:331-345, 1888, 21.*

116. Koffka, K.: *The growth of the mind.* Harcourt, Brace, Co. New York, 1925, 3.*
117. Kogerer, H.: Worttaubheit, Melodientaubheit, Gebärdenagnosie. *Ztschr. Neur.u.Psychiat., 92*:469, 1924, 20.*
118. Köhler, W.: Akustische Untersuchungen. *Ztschr.Psychol., 72*:1, 1915, 21.*
119. Kramer, F.: Beiträge zur Lehre von der Alexie und der amnestischen Aphasie. *Mschr.f.Psychiat.u.Neur., 68*:346-360, 1928, 16.*
120. Kroh, O.: *Subjektive Anschauungsbilder der Jugendlichen.* Gottingen, 1922.
121. Kuenberg, M von.: Über das Erfassen einfacher Beziehungen an anschaulichen Material bei Hirngeschädigten insbesondere bei Aphasischen. *Ztschr.f.Neur.u.Psychiat., 85*:120-163, 1923, 22.*
122. Kussmaul, A.: *Die Störungen der Sprache.* Vogel, Leipzig, 1885, 10, 15.*
123. Ladame, P. and Monakow, C. von: Observation d'aphémie pure (anarthrie corticale). *Encéphale, 3*:193-228, 1908, 4.*
124. Lewandowsky, M.: Über Abspaltung des Farbensinnes. *Mschr.f.Psychiat. u.Neur., 23*:488-510, 1908, 3.*
125. Lewin, K.: Das Problem der Willensmessung und der Assoziation. *Psychol. Forsch., 1*:191-302, 1922; *2*:65-140, 1922.
126. Leyser, E.: Die zentralen Dysarthrien und ihre Pathogenese. *Berl.klin. Wschr., 2*:2176, 1923, 4.*
127. Liepmann, H.: Ein Fall von Echolalie. *Neur.Zbl., 19*:389-399, 1900.
128. Liepmann, H.: *Ein Fall von reiner Worttaubheit.* Berlin, 1908, 15.
129. Liepmann, H.: *Drei Aufsätze aus dem Apraxiegebeit.* S. Karger, Berlin, 1908.
130. Liepmann, H.: Zum Stande der Aphasiefrage. *Neur.Zbl., 28*:449-484, 1909, 15.*
131. Liepmann, H.: Motor aphasia, anarthria, and apraxia. *Trans. 17th. Internat'l. Cong. Med.,* London, pp. 97-115, 1913.
132. Long: Un cas d'aphasie par lesion de l'hemisphere gauche chez un gauchier. *Encéphale,* 520, 1913, 8.*
133. Lotmar, F.: Zur Kenntnis der erschwerten Wortfindung und ihrer Bedeutung für das Denken des Aphasischen. *Schweiz.Arch.Neur.u. Psychiat., 5*:206-239, 1919, 3, 22.*
134. Lotmar, F. and Montet, C.: *Rev. neurol., 14*:22, 1906.
135. Maas, O.: Uber Agrammatismus und die Bedeutung der rechten Hemisphare fur die Sprache. *Neur.Zbl., 39*:465-488, 506-511, 1920, 14.*
136. Mann, L.: Kasuistische Beiträge zur Hirnchirurgie und Hirnlokalisation. *Mschr.Psychiat., 4*:369, 1898, 21.*
137. Mann, M.: Ein Fall von motorischer Amusie. *Neur. Zbl., 36*:149, 1917.
138. Margulies: Studien über Echographie (Pick). *Mschr.f.Psychiat.u.Neur., 22*:479-490, 1907.
139. Marie, P.: Révision det la question de l'aphasie. *Sem.Méd., 21*:241-247, 493-500, 565-571, 1906, 22.*

140. Marie, P.: Rectifications á propos de la question de l' aphasie. *Presse Méd., 4*:25, 1907, 22.*
141. Markus, H.: Sensorische Paramnesie. *Ztschr.f.Neur.u.Psychiat., 81*:625, 1923, 21.*
142. Mazurkiewicz: Störungen der Gebärdensprache. *Jahrb.Neur., 19*:524, 1900, 20.*
143. Mendel, K.: Über Rechtshirnigkeit bei Rechtshändern. *Neur.Zbl., 131*: 156, 1912; *33*:291, 1914, 8.*
144. Mendel, K.: Motorisch Amusie. *Neur.Zbl., 35*:354, 1916, 21.*
145. Meringer, R. and Mayer, K.: *Versprechen und Verlesen. Eine psychologisch-linguistische Studie.* Stuttgart, 1895.
146. Messer, K.: Experimentelle-psychologische Untersuchungen über das Denken. *Arch.f.Psychol., 8*:1-224, 1906.
147. Messmer, O.: *Zur Psychologie des Lesens bei Kindern und Erwachsenen.* Inaug. Diss. Univ. Zurich, Engelmann, Leipzig, 1903.
148. Meumann, E.: *Die Enstehung der ersten Wortbedeutungen beim Kinde.* Leipzig, 1908, 3.*
149. Mills, C.: Aphasia and the cerebral zone of speech. *Am.J.Med.Sci., 128*: 375-393, 1904, 15.*
150. Mirallie, C.: *De l'aphasie sensorielle.* These de Paris, 1896, 15.*
151. Misch, W. and Frankl. K.: Beiträg zur Alexielehre. *Mschr.f.Psychiat.u. Neur., 71*:1-47, 1929, 16.*
152. Monakow, C. von: *Gehirnpathologie.* Halder, Vienna, 1905, 1.*
153. Monakow, C. von: *Die Lokalisation im Grosshirn und der Abbau der Funktion durch kortikale Herde.* Bergmann, Weisbaden, 1914, 1, 8.*
154. Moutier, F.: *L'aphasie de Broca.* Steinheil, Paris, 1908, 4.*
155. Naville, F.: Mémorie d'un médecin aphasique. *Arch. de Psychol., 17*:1-57, 1918, 16, 22.*
156. Oppenheim, H.: *Lehrbuch der Nervenkrankheiten.* S. Karger, Berlin, 1902.
157. Osborne: *Dubl.J.Med. and Chem.Sci., 4*:157, 1834, 10.*
158. Peretti: Über Speigelschrift. *Berl.klin.Wschr.,* 477, 1882.
159. Peritz, G.: Zur Pathopsychologie des Rechnents. *Dtsch.Z.Nervenheilk., 61*:234-340, 1918, 18.*
160. Peters, W.: Zur Entwicklung der Farbenwahrnehmung nach Versuchen an abnormen Kindern. *Psychol. Forschr., 3*:150, 1915.
161. Peters, W.: *Münch.Med.Wschr.,* p. 1116, 1908.
162. Pick, A.: Mitteilungen aus der psychiatrischen Klinik. *Prag.Med.Wschr.,* pp. 25-27, 1891.
163. Pick, A.: Zur Lehre von der Dyslexie. *Neur.Zbl.,* Vol. 5, 1891.
164. Pick, A.: Beiträge zur Lehre von den Störungen der Sprache. *Archiv.f. Psychiat.u.Neur., 23*:896-918, 1892, 11.*
165. Pick, A.: *Beiträge zur Pathologie und pathologischen Anatomie des Centralnervensystems.* S. Karger, Berlin, 1898, 14.*
166. Pick, A.: Sur l'echographie. *Rev. neurol.,* p. 822, 1900.

167. Pick, A.: Über die Bedeutung des akustischen Sprachzentrums als Hemmungsorgan des Sprachmechanismus. *37*:823, 1900, 10.*
168. Pick, A.: Zur Symptomatologie der linksseitigen Schläfenlappenatrophie *Mschr.f.Psychiat.u.Neur., 16*:378, 1904, 13.*
169. Pick, A.: Über sprachlichen Infantilismus als Folge cerebraler Herderkrankung bei Erwachsenen. *J.Abnorm.Soc.Psycol.*, Vol. 50, 1906.
170. Pick, A.: Zuz Analyse der Elemente der Amusie und deren Vorkommen im Rahmen aphasischen Störungen. *Mschr.f.Psychiat.u.Neur., 8*:87, 1906, 21.*
171. Pick, A.: *Forensische Bedeutung der Aphasien. Handb.d.arztl.Sachverständigentätigkeit.* Braumüller, Wien u. Leipzig, 1909, 22.*
172. Pick, A.: *Über das Sprachverständnis.* Barth, Leipzig, 1909, 5, 10, 12, 15.*
173. Pick, A.: *Die agrammatischen Sprachstörungen.* Springer, Berlin, 1913, 6, 7, 14.*
174. Pick, A.: Über das Verhältnis von Echolalie und Nachsprechen. *Mschr.f.Psychiat.u.Neur., 39*:65, 1916, 12.*
175. Pick, A.: Zur Frage nach der Natur der Echolalie. *Psychol.Forschr., 4*:1, 1916.
176. Pick, A.: Über das Verhältnis zwischen motorischer und sensorischer Sprachregion. *Archiv.f.Psychiat.u.Neur., 56*:810, 1916, 10.*
177. Pick, A.: Über Spiegelsprache und ihre nahestehende Erscheinungen. *Zschr.f.d.ges.Neur.u.Psychiat., 42*:325, 1918.
178. Pick, A.: Über Änderungen des Sprachcharakters als Begleiterscheinung aphasischer Störungen. *Ztschr.f.d.ges.Neur.u.Psychiat., 45*:230, 1919.
179. Pick, A.: *Die neurologische Forschungsrichtung in der Psychopathologie.* S. Karger, Berlin, 1921.
180. Pick, A.: Sprachpsychologie und andere Studien zur Aphasielehre. *Schweiz. Arch.f.Neur.u.Psychiat., 12*:105-135, 1923.
181. Piéron, H.: Le notion des centres coordinateurs cérébraux et la méchanisme du langage. *Rev. Philos., 46*:271, 1921, 1.*
182. Pitres, A.: Considerations sur l'agraphie (agraphie motrice pure). *Rev. Méd., 4*:855-873, 1884, 17.*
183. Pitres, A.: *L'aphasie amnestique et ses variétés cliniques.* Alcan, Paris, 1898, 13.*
184. Pitres, A.: Études sur les paraphasies. *Rev. de Med.*, pp. 337, 549, 1899, 10, 12.*
185. Poppelreuter, W.: Über den Versuch einer Revision der psychophysiologischen Lehre von der elementaren Assoziation und Reproduktion. *Mschr.f.Psychiat.u.Neur., 37*:278, 1915, 6.*
186. Poppelreuter, W.: *Die psychischen Schädigungen durch Kopfschuss im Kriege.*, 2 vol. Voss, Leipzig, 1914-1917, 18.*
187. Pötzl, O.: *Zur Klinik und Anatomie der reinen Wortaubheit.* S. Karger, Berlin, 1919, 15.*
188. Pötzl, O.: Über die Herderscheinungen bei Läsionen des linken hinteren Schläfenlappen. *Med.Klin., 19*:7-11, 1923.

189. Quensel, F.: Über Erscheinungen und Grundlagen der Worttaubheit. *Dtsch.Z.Nervenheilk., 35*:25, 1908, 15.*
190. Quensel, F.: Über transkortikale motorische Aphasie. *Mschr.f.Psychiat.u. Neur., 26*:286, 1909.
191. Quensel, F. and Pfeiffer, R.: Über reine sensorische Amusie. *Ztschr.f.d. ges.Neur.u.Psychiat., 81*:311-330, 1923, 21.*
192. Redlich, E.: Über die sogennante subcortikale Alexie.. *Jahrb.Psychiat.u. Neur., 13*:243-302, 1895, 16.*
193. Righetti: *Riv.Pat.Nerv.,* 1900.
194. Rohardt: Ein Fall von motorischer Amusie. *Neur.Zbl.,* Vol. 38, 1919, 21.*
195. Saint-Paul, G.: *Le langage interieur et les paraphasies (la fonction endophasique).* Paris, 1904, 7.*
196. Salomon, E.: Motorische Aphasie mit Agrammatismus und sensorisch-agrammatischen Störungen. *Mschr.f.Psychiat.u.Neur., 35*:181-275, 1914.
197. Schuster, P.: Beiträge zur Kenntnis der Alexie. *Mschr.f.Psychiat.u.Neur., 25*:349-424, 1909, 16.*
198. Selz, O.: *Zur Psychologie des produktiven Denkens,* etc. Cohen, Bonn, 1922, 6.*
199. Sherrington, C.: *The Integrative Action of the Nervous System.* Yale University Press, New Haven, 1906, 9.*
200. Sittig, O.: Über Störung des Ziffernschreibens bei Aphasischen. *Ztschr.f. Pathopsychol., 3*:298-306, 1919, 18.*
201. Sittig, O.: Störung des Ziffernschreibens und Rechnens bei einem Hirnverletzten. *Mschr.Psychiat.u.Neur., 49*:299, 1921, 18.*
202. Solder: Über Perseveration, eine formale Störung im Vorstellungsablaufe. *Jahrb.Psychiat., 18*:479, 1899, 11.*
203. Stauffenberg, J. von: Klinische und anatomische Beiträge zur Kenntnis der aphasischen, agnostischen und apraktischen Symptome. *Ztschr.f.d. ges. Neur.u.Psychiat., 39*:71-213, 1918, 13.*
204. Stern, C. and Stern, W.: *Die Kindersprache.* Leipzig, 1907, 3.*
205. Stertz, G.: Die klinische Stellung der amnestischen und transcorticalen motorischen Aphasie. *Dtsch.Z Nervenheilk., 51*:239, 1914, 13.*
206. Stier: *Untersuchungen über Linkshadigkeit und die funktionellen Differenzen der Hirnhalften,* 1911.
207. Stransky, E.: *Über Sprachverwirrtheit.* Marhold, Halle, 1905.
208. Stumpf, C.: *Die Sprachlaute,* Berlin, 1926, 15.*
209. Teufer, J.: *Die Symptomenbilder der Amusie, ihre Psychologie und ihre Untersuchung.* Beiträge zur Anatomie, Physiologie, Pathologie, und Therapie des Ohres, der Nase, und des Halses. *20*:149, 1924, 21.*
210. Thiele, R.: Aphasie, Apraxie, Agnosie. In O. Bumke (Ed.): *Handb.d. Geisteskrankh.* Springer, Berlin, 1928, vol. 2, pp. 243-365, 1.*
211. Vernet, P. and Merland, A.: Un cas d'aphasie totale. *Bull. de la Soc.clin. de méd.ment., 10*:230-234, 1922.
212. Verworn: *Ztschr.allg.Physiol., 6*:118, 1907.

213. Wernicke, C.: *Der aphasische Symptomenkomplex.* Cohn and Weigert, Breslau, 1874, 10, 15, 16.*
214. Wernicke, C.: *Grundiss der Psychiatrie.* Barth. Leipzig, 1900, 22.*
215. Wernicke, C.: Ein Fall von isolierter Agraphie. *Mschr.Psychiat.u.Neur., 13*:241-265, 1903, 17.*
216. Wilks, S.: *Guy's Hosp. Rep.,* Vol. 24, 1879.
217. Woerkom, W. van: Über Störungen im Denken bei Aphasiepatienten. *Mschr.f.Psychiat.u.Neur., 59*:256-322, 1925, 22.*
218. Wolff, G.: *Klinische und kritische Beiträge zur Lehre von den Sprachstörungen.,* 1904, 13.*
219. Wündt, W.: *Völkerpsychologie.* Engelmann, Leipzig, 1928, 20.*
220. Wurtzen: Einzelne Formen der Amusie, durch Beispiele erlautert. *Dtsch. Z.Nervenheilk., 24*:465, 1903, 21.*